Back Talk

Back Talk

HOW TO DIAGNOSE AND CURE LOW BACK PAIN AND SCIATICA

Loren Fishman, M.D., and
Carol Ardman

W. W. Norton & Company
New York London

For information about permission to reproduce selections from this book, write to
Permissions, W. W. Norton & Company, Inc., 500 Fifth Avenue, New York, NY 10110.

The text of this book is composed in Dante
with the display set in Bembo
Composition and Manufacturing by The Haddon Craftsmen, Inc.
Book design by Chris Welch

Library of Congress Cataloging-in-Publication Data
Fishman, Loren.
Back talk: how to diagnose and cure low back pain and sciatica / by Loren
Fishman and Carol Ardman.
p.   cm.
Includes index.
ISBN 0-393-04129-8
1. Backache—Popular works.   2. Sciatica—Popular works.   I. Ardman, Carol.
II. Title.
RD771.B217F568   1997
617.5'64—dc21   97-426
CIP

W. W. Norton & Company, Inc., 500 Fifth Avenue, New York, N.Y. 10110
http://www.wwnorton.com

W. W. Norton & Company Ltd., 10 Coptic Street, London WC1A 1PU

1 2 3 4 5 6 7 8 9 0

FOR JOSH, ALEX, AND RACHEL

Contents

Acknowledgments

Thanks go to Mark Thomas, M.D., for his patience and fortitude in reviewing the manuscript for this book, and to Todd Olsen, Ph.D., for taking time to share his knowledge of anatomy with us. For their generous help we also wish to acknowledge Ivan Strausz, M.D., Heinz Lippmann, M.D., Stanley Wainapel, M.D., Barry Pinchoff, M.D., and Yoga teachers Ellen Saltonstall and Victor Oppenheimer.

Vaune Hatch punctually and efficiently executed our ideas for illustrations.

We are grateful to Jill Bialosky, Susan Middleton, Ellen Levine, Eileen Stukane, and Anne Nevins. Joyce Wadler stimulated our thinking before we began to put words on paper. Flor Salas and Vanessa Aldebot provided us with a warm, supportive working environment.

Author's Note

The information in this book is meant to help you identify the cause of your back pain. Of course, only a doctor or other professional can provide a definitive diagnosis.

Behind Your Backache

For many of the 150 million Americans who suffer from chronic or acute low back pain, searching for relief isn't only a necessity; it's also a hobby. No wonder. Back pain is mysterious and perverse. It often strikes for no apparent reason and lasts for weeks or months. And, of course, it hurts. Even a relatively mild attack of backache can prevent an otherwise healthy person from accomplishing something as simple as getting out of bed.

Coping with low back pain is practically a national pastime, and one that wastes an incredible amount of time and money. After the common cold, backache is the single greatest cause of missed days of work. The pain so many people feel racks up an estimated $20 billion to $50 billion a year. Yet 60 percent of back pain disappears spontaneously, never to return. Another 20 to 30 percent can be cured without spending a dime, just by making some small nonmedical adjustment, like changing the height of a desk chair or losing 10 pounds. All in all, an astounding 65 to 85 percent of all back pain vanishes without any treatment or is easily relieved!

Then why the sale of tons of over-the-counter analgesics? Obviously people don't hesitate to dose themselves with these medications when backache hits. Also, statistics prove that the vast majority of doctors, no matter what their specialty, recommend these over-the-counter painkillers before any other treatment, because they reduce both pain and inflammation.

If pain is relieved, why do hordes of supplicants rush to an ever-changing flock of specialists and quacks? Some observers might write it off to social trends or fads. As a physician who has been treating back pain for fifteen years, I believe the real answer is less complicated. Without correctly identifying the cause of a pain in the back, no rational solution, medical or nonmedical, can be put into effect.

It's not just the doctor who benefits from knowing the cause of an individual's backache. I believe a patient needs this information as much as or more than any health-care worker. There are many reasons for this, not the least of which is that patients who understand the cause of their pain make faster and more complete recoveries.

Another crucial reason victims of backache must share the responsibility for their own diagnosis and cure is that it's necessary for successfully negotiating the world of health maintenance organizations (HMOs). To take advantage of "allotted" visits and cogently argue for a specialist, diagnostic test, or other treatment, you as the patient must have information about your own condition. It's up to you, the person whose back hurts, to discover the facts and participate in subsequent treatment decisions.

Unfortunately your need to understand the nature of the problem is tricky. An ironic rule characterizes back pain: making the proper diagnosis is almost invariably more difficult than achieving a cure.

An accurate diagnosis—which can spring from such a seemingly insignificant observation as the fact that the heel of one shoe is more worn down than the other—is crucial to alleviating back pain. Even an experienced specialist might miss the quirk in an individual's walk that has been stabbing the person in the back for years. But almost as soon as something like a gait irregularity is spotted, it can be corrected. On the whole, conditions that elude diagnosis are often easily remedied once the cause is found, while the more serious problems—those quickly turned up by a CT scan or an MRI—are harder to manage and cure.

Sciatica complicates all this. The sometimes excruciating electric shocklike pain that travels down the leg is the worst part for 35 to 40 percent of people who have chronic or intermittent back pain. It's the culprit in 95 percent of back pain that puts people on the operating table. Though sciatica is a symptom of a number of different conditions, it almost always accompanies severe backache and can occur in any intensity by itself.

The medical establishment currently tends to lump sciatica into the general category of back pain rather than treating it as a separate problem or a significant symptom of something else. I think misunderstanding and misinterpretation result from not giving sciatica its due as an affliction with its own identity and origins, which are as diverse as uterine fibroid tumors, a herniated ("slipped") disk, and piriformis syndrome (See the Glossary for definitions of these and other terms.)

With or without sciatica, even slight low back pain can make the victim unable to bend low enough to pick up a briefcase or tie a shoe. And if the ache doesn't make the patient crazy, deciding how to seek a cure just might. Which works better, ice or heat, exercise or bed rest? Should the patient see an orthopedist, a physiatrist (a doctor of physical medicine and rehabilitation), a chiropractor, an acupuncturist, a massage therapist, or a psychiatrist?

This book is devoted to helping you answer those questions and many others. I hope the information will be valuable in helping you with the task of getting rid of your backache or keeping it under control.

The Chinese have a parable, which applies to all goals, including curing back pain. It's the story of people using different paths to reach the identical destination. So a person with a muscle spasm, for example, might be able to just wait it out. Or she might get relief from the family doctor's prescription for muscle relaxant, massage, and heat. The same individual might be able to conquer the ache with a single visit to a physical therapist. I believe knowledge will aid you in your choice of a route and will speed you on your way to a cure.

Back Talk

CHAPTER 1

The Spine

A woman once sat on the other side of my desk and said, "It hurts, but don't waste your time explaining the technical part. I've never been any good at science. I go blank when doctors haul out their anatomy models. Just tell me what's wrong and I'll do whatever's necessary to fix it."

That woman wasn't giving herself a chance. I have found that with even a little encouragement most patients, instead of being daunted by anatomical and scientific information for which they may have no background, can comprehend all the medical information they need. They become anatomists eager to examine the skeleton I keep in the corner, as well as to look with me at their X rays and other diagnostic tests. This curiosity stimulates patients to take pleasure in acquiring basic education about how their bodies function, and it serves them well in the process of working with their doctors toward a cure. Then it becomes their strongest ally in preventing further dysfunction or pain.

An elementary understanding of the spine and its related structures is necessary not only for those patients who don't have a diagnosis, but also for those who know what's wrong. It's not that patients can't get relief from pain or stay pain-free without detailed knowledge of how their bodies work—only that those goals are more easily met and sustained with an educated patient who has some idea of the actual physical process of trying to achieve a cure.

The Spine and Civilization

Until something goes wrong, most of us take our spines for granted. Yet the physical abilities of every creature in the animal kingdom, from amoebas to sharks to humans, depend on the presence or absence of a spine. Possessing a real backbone makes the difference between bounding across the African veldt or crawling like an inchworm—between a person performing the precise movements of a pirouette or a starfish scuttling across the ocean floor.

Our prehistoric ancestors lived in water. It took millennia for the processes of evolution to transform their masses of cartilage and toughened fibers into bones. Fins and wings appeared, then arms and legs, and eventually hands and feet. All these evolutionary changes made it possible for our precursors to move out of the water and support themselves on land. For us, further modifications placed locomotion in the lower part of our bodies, leaving the upper limbs free to hold and manipulate objects.

As vertebrates, we humans and a vast number of other animals, including fish and turtles, are the same in that we share the characteristic of having a central nervous system. But the particular aspects of the human backbone, including the brain, also differentiate us from other animals, allowing us purposeful movements like walking upright. The rest of our bones make a difference too. No creatures but vertebrates have bones at all. We, using our bones as levers and poles, can actually thrust ourselves forward, grasping things firmly and moving freely, even vaulting through the air with precision of movement. None of this could happen without the stiffness and jointedness of bones associated with a strong but flexible spine.

Bones in general and the spine in particular provide both leverage and the ability to move with accuracy. The rigidity of a bone makes it possible for a muscle to contract at one place to produce a particular movement at another. Flexibility—poised, bending, refined movement—is created by the way bones fit together at joints. Flexibility helps us adjust to changes in position, even to shock. The curves of the spine, its disks, joints, supportive musculature, and connective tissue all make the spine strong enough for a fire fighter to carry a man out of a burning building. If that fire fighter has to jump down to the street from a height of several feet, the flexible spine acts as a spring, returning him or her to an original upright position quickly and without injury.

It's amazing to contemplate what bones and the spine have meant for human beings. In addition to giving us the ability to stand upright and therefore to walk, they allow us to present ourselves to each other chiefly front to front. Thanks to our anatomy we can carry things and bring food to our lips with our hands. We don't have to carry things in our mouths but can use them to speak.

The spine, with its combination of stability at the ribs and flexibility at both jointed ends (Figure 1), with the extraordinary developments of head and legs at top and bottom, has promoted our ability to perform complicated, diverse, powerful, and detailed movements. All this leads me to conclude that the spine is a significant factor in the rise of civilization.

A General Look at the Anatomy of the Spine

The spine (Figure 2) is made up of seven elements: bones, muscles and nerves, which are held together by tendons, ligaments, disks, and other connective tissue. Tensions created by all these parts against the spine keep us erect, much the way ropes and wires, all pulling downward, keep a tent pole vertical. The interactions among these elements both shape our bodies and let them move at will.

Massive architecture characterizes the lower part of the backbone

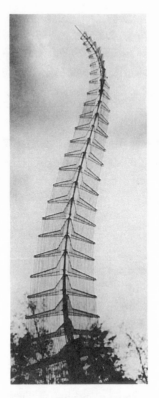

Figure 1. Flexible Column, by Frei Otto (1963).

and our hip joints. The pelvis connects the hip joints to the spine at the sacrum. These bones and the legs that attach to them are big enough to support and stabilize the vertical column of the body. Up near the neck, at the other end of the spinal cord, the joints thicken and the bones get thinner and smaller. This allows for mobility and flexibility and gives us the capacity for speedily directing the organs of sense, which are chiefly located in our heads.

The same type of arrangement—bigger at the bottom and smaller at the top—exists with the structures that hold up the spine. Down low, large muscles direct and power the movements of our legs and our trunks and compensate for the physical stress these actions cause within the spine. Here's an example of physical stress: amazingly, the apparently simple, unathletic act of sitting down produces about 528 pounds of force per square inch on a lumbar spinal disk. If you lifted a 2,000-pound suitcase by its handle, you'd feel a similar pressure on your palm.

Farther up the back, smaller muscles control our arms and head in their complex movements. These also undergo terrific stress while performing even routine duties, like buttering a piece of bread or bending to sniff the aroma of a flower. According to the position of the lower body, movements with the upper part of the back can put us "way out on a limb." Frequently the muscles higher up can't compensate for what we're doing with the muscles farther down. In the common situation—for example, when wriggling into tight blue jeans—abnormal stress on the lower back can cause upper back pain.

LEVERAGE

One of the main jobs of the spine is to provide leverage for the contracting muscles so that we can move at will. When you look at the placement of the network of spinal bones, the way we humans use leverage becomes apparent. It's leverage that accounts for the tremendous speed at which the baseball can be thrown, the balance achieved by a circus high-wire walker, the ability of a 110-pound mother to toss around her 30-pound toddler. But while leverage is a natural advantage that we use to accomplish seemingly impossible tasks, it also has disadvantages.

Because of leverage, when your right hand picks up a 10-pound package, the force exerted on the bones and muscles on the left side of your spine can amount to more than 100 pounds! In other words, when it comes to leverage and the spine, slightly miscalculating the weight of a frying pan, for instance, or stepping unexpectedly into a depression in the pavement under your foot, or leaning over the wrong way when adjusting the car seat, can be multiplied many times. An unconscious or automatic "mistake" like the ones just mentioned can magnify the stress on a muscle, tendon, or ligament to the point of injury.

SEGMENTATION AND SUPPORT

Instead of being one long single bone with a joint at either end, like the arm's humerus between the shoulder and elbow, our spines are made up of many small bones with joints throughout. This highly specialized but versatile structure supports our weight, cushions forces like a spring, holds us erect, and adjusts to a vast number of positions.

Without the muscles that symmetrically support it, the spine would tumble to the floor. The symmetry may appear to be in one dimension, from side to side, but length and depth must also be considered. Each vertebra exerts a similar force and imposes limits on the vertebrae below and above it (Figure 2).

The basic modular units of the spine—the "bricks" of which the entire structure is built—are each composed of two adjacent spinal vertebrae, the disk between them, and their associated nerve roots. Each vertebra is therefore part of two vertebral units: the one below it (with the nerve root and disk between) and the one above it with that nerve root and disk. These units, acting in an overlapping series, produce flexibility by distributing the bending, tilting, and twisting movements of which each is capable. For example, if each of the twenty-four vertebrae (excluding the sacrum, and coccyx, which are rigid) were to rotate 4 degrees, the total rotation would amount to more than 90 degrees and would bring the torso to the position of a baseball player who has just completed the swing of a bat.

The spine, supported by muscles, tendons, ligaments, and connective tissue, resembles a collapsible tent pole. Another way to look at the human body is as a tensegrity—a stable but dynamic three-dimensional structure whose elements, under tension, help the whole to keep its form. The spine is also reminiscent of the keystone in a Roman arch, which focuses forces from right and left, balancing them

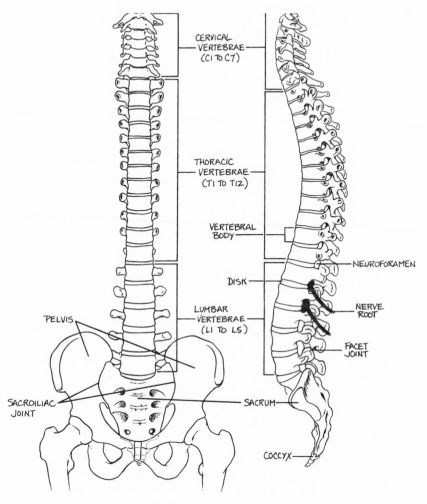

Figure 2. The human spine.

and keeping the entire structure of the body aloft. The spine could also be compared to the segmented transmitting antenna of a radio station with the many guy wires that hold it up in a vertical position, each with its slanting but relatively equal *downward* force.

At the same time, movement is intrinsic to the functioning of the spine. People bend, twist, and tilt in all directions. It is during these movements that many painful injuries occur.

Individual Bones—The 34 Bones of the Spine

THE FOUNDATION

Let's start at the bottom and work up (Figure 3). The coccyx consists of three to five fused bones at the base of the back that don't move relative to each other. We commonly call this series the tailbone—in animals with four legs, such as cats or monkeys, it has many more segments than ours and *is* a tail. Some animals, of course use their tails to maintain balance. Because we have to balance without this handy appendage, there is more stress on our spines. At times when we can't keep our balance and fall, the human coccyx can break, producing a condition called coccygodynia, which we'll go into later.

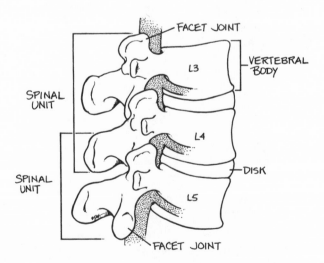

Figure 3. The spine owes its flexible strength to overlapping units.

The next five bones up the ladder are also fused. They make up another single bone called the sacrum. The sacrum is a spade-shaped bone that fits between the two halves of the pelvis. It is positioned just below the small of the back, where the arch of the lumbar spine actually ends.

I must digress at this point to discuss structures related to the spine but not part of the spine itself. The sacrum is housed between the two halves of the pelvis, which is the only place the spine connects to the lower limbs. The iliac bones, which make up the outer part of each side of the pelvis, fit into the sacroiliac joints. These joints are the large, saddle-shaped interfaces between the sides of the pelvis and the sacrum. It's in this area that abnormalities and asymmetries (imbalances) frequently cause pain in the lower back.

The sacroiliac joints differ from other joints. They're thicker and move only a few millimeters. Though their relative immobility makes them resistant to gravitational forces, they're subject to the tremendous stresses and strains created by the large levers of the lower extremities and trunk and the long extension of the upper extremities. The sacroiliac joints are also unusual in that some of the most powerful muscles in the body arch over them.

In a sense, the sacroiliac joints are the crossroads of four powerful forces. First, they support the trunk, shoulders, arms, and head in every position. We can bend our flexible spines to increase pressure or to cushion the forces on the sacroiliac joints. Second, the joints are the center of locomotive activity, including walking, running, and stopping abruptly. So if you walk and swing your arms, carry a briefcase and hail a taxi, or hold someone in your arms and dance, the upper and lower extremity forces meet and result in movement at the sacroiliac joint. Third, these joints are subject to gravity, which is not always equally applied, so they must be strong and flexible. And last, in women these joints must withstand the birth process, where the baby's head must pass close to the L5-S1 vertebral unit.[1]

[1]Clinically the vertebral bones of the back are identified by letter and number, in this case, L5 (for fifth lumbar) and S1 (for first sacral).

LUMBAR SPINE

The part of the back known as the lumbar spine almost always has five large, distinct vertebrae.[2]

These vertebral bones rest upon vertebral disks, complex structures of connective tissue that contain no nerves or blood vessels. The disks separate the vertebrae by about three-quarters of an inch.

Each vertebra has two facets that come out of the top like arms and two more that descend from the bottom like legs. The four facets are loosely joined to their counterpart facets in the vertebrae above and below (see Figure 2 on page 25). When the facets slide across each other, the lumbar spine moves, vertebra by vertebra, producing the basic forward-and-back motion familiar in fast dancing, sex, arching exercises, and other activities that produce a big belly with a pushed-out bottom, or a tilted pelvis and a pulled-in bottom. When viewed from the side the lumbar spine is concave relative to the back of the body, or, in medical terms, lordotic.

Because it's too low to benefit from reinforcement by the ribs, this area of the spine can get into trouble when bending from side to side, forward and backward, and also when twisting. The leverages and amount of weight this area must withstand are the greatest of any along the entire spine. Below is firm stability; above is fast, strong activity. The lumbar spine must resolve these contrary influences with a combination of strength and flexibility.

Like the center point of a bridge, this is the part of the back under the most strain and with the fewest resources for support. Support, however, does come from a cylindrical girdle of muscles surrounding the body at the abdomen and helping to keep the body erect. These muscles brace us as the ribs do, but flexibly rather than with the rigidity of bone.

---

[2]In rare cases there are six vertebrae, and sometimes there are four and a half. This latter situation, called a hemivertebra or absent vertebra, can cause serious mechanical damage and pain.

THORACIC SPINE

The 12 vertebrae that have ribs attached are called the thoracic spine. The function of the ribs is to hold a space open in the body, creating a partial vacuum for inflating the lungs. They also protect the backbone and the vital organs—the heart, lungs and liver. The ribs exert a great deal of leverage against this long, flexible column of bones. The upper nine ribs arise from the spine and are joined at the front like a clasped purse. They allow the spine only a little motion. When looked at from the side, this part of the back is slightly concave relative to the front of the body, or kyphotic.

The lower three ribs are like an open purse. They don't enclose anything, but they are protective, and they allow for more motion than the first nine ribs. The joints between the last thoracic vertebra and the first lumbar vertebra (that is, between T12 and L1) allow these relatively immobile regions to rotate from side to side. These are the joints that let a seated driver turn to judge distances when parking. Since so much turning is centered on these joints, they are subject to a lot of wear and tear, and are often where pathology like osteoarthritis (degenerative joint disease) begins.

CERVICAL SPINE

The uppermost part of the backbone, the cervical spine, has seven vertebrae. Like a medieval tower, these vertebrae get progressively smaller as they ascend toward the head. Their joints are broad, nearly horizontal, and slope gently upward toward the front of the body. They aren't fused like the sacrum, nor do they have any rigid outer supports like the ribs, and therefore are capable of a great deal of motion. The neck, for instance, can turn 90 degrees in either direction, the ear can almost lie on the shoulder, and the head can rear backwards until it's almost horizontal.

Our brains respond to outside stimulation even before we know it, and nature has sculpted the top of the spine for flexibility so that we can point our ears, eyes, noses, and mouths toward interesting objects or events. The anatomy of the uppermost reaches of the spine has yet another advantage: it supports the large, symmetrical structure of the skull.

In a sense, the fixed bones of the skull are the antithesis of the fixed bones at the other end of the spine—the sacrum and coccyx. After all, the head's function is to house the brain, not to do much physical labor. While the work of the brain is to transmit impulses, the role of the sacrum and coccyx—which are flat, not hollow—is to transmit forces. Nevertheless, the pelvis also houses vital organs.

The head is the site of attachment of many muscles important for its support and for balanced movement of arms, shoulders, and the cervical, thoracic, and lumbar spine. We tailless bipeds use our heads to cantilever forces, keep our balance, and compensate for low back pain. That's why headache and cervical spine pain frequently accompany or follow episodes of low back pain.

Muscles and Nerves

Generally speaking, muscles provide locomotion by wielding the pressure that moves the bones. But the gravity exerted by the earth and the leverages involved between the muscles and the bones must also be taken into consideration when we think about how human beings move or change position. The spine normally affords a means for muscles to support structures on the other side of the body for asymmetrical activities, like taking clothes off a line or hammering a nail. Of course, symmetrical muscles also allow us to maneuver ourselves symmetrically, as we do when we stand, walk or swim the breaststroke.

Any time muscles move something, they contract. But muscles don't just contract. They also absorb shock and release their tension in a controlled way. An example is walking. When the heel makes contact with the pavement, the rest of the foot smoothly follows it. Controlled muscle release lets the knees bend slowly, for example, when you take a seat in the theater.

Inside the spine there are two kinds of nerves, motor and sensory. Motor nerves transmit impulses originating in the brain and spinal cord down to the muscles and glands. These are the nerves that initiate movement. Sensory nerves bring messages from the joints, muscles, organs, blood vessels, and skin up to the brain. They provide information about what's outside ourselves and about what we're doing.

Together one nerve fiber and the muscle fiber it activates are called a motor unit. Normally, one fiber is unable to act without the other. Injury to the nerve can cause either involuntary, intense contraction (spasm), or weakness or paralysis (not enough contraction). Both too much contraction and too little can cause pain. Spasm overstimulates sensory nerve fibers and undernourishes muscle fibers; weak muscles can overstretch and sustain structural damage.

So when it comes to back pain, you need the sensory nerves to give you feedback about whether that muscle is doing its job correctly. If the feedback loop doesn't work properly, the common result is spasm, sprain, strain, and/or minor joint misalignments. (I will describe these conditions later.)

Tendons and Ligaments

Both tendons and ligaments are made of a type of tissue called collagen; These structures are usually round, and tough like leather thongs. The difference between tendons and ligaments is that tendons connect muscles to bones allowing muscles, when they contract, to move the bones. Ligaments connect bone to bone around joints and keep the bones at a relatively constant distance, whether or not they're moving.

With few exceptions, tendons connect muscles to bones. There is a tendon at each end of every muscle. Tendons exert "pull" on the bones, sometimes moving them, sometimes holding them firmly in place. Tendons can slow you down or steady you when you need stability. Through their tendons, muscles in your back exert just a little less force than gravity, so they slowly lengthen when you bend down smoothly (eccentric contraction) to get into position to tie your shoe. When you've reached your shoelace, the muscles and tendons exert a force that equals gravity to keep your body in place (isometric contraction). Then muscles pull the tendons to move your fingers so that they can manipulate the shoelaces (concentric contraction).

We get into trouble when something—an accident or developments that occur with aging, for instance—makes muscles and their tendons unable to perform their proper function. A tendon shouldn't stretch to the point of fraying or breaking, nor should it compress a nerve that happens to run under or above it, or constantly rub against a bursa (a soft pouch between a tendon and a bone that protects each from the other). Tendons contain sensory nerves that will inhibit muscles when the pull on the tendon is too strong.

Ligaments hold bones together from standard locations at their ends. Just as muscles cause bones to move relative to one another, ligaments keep them at the correct distance from one another. Ligaments become a problem when they're inflamed, torn, or strained. For instance, if a house painter always holds the paint pail with the left hand and makes brush strokes with the right hand, he or she might stretch the ligaments on the right side of the spine, causing pain.

Disks

Rather than joining vertebrae, disks separate them. These highly structured elements of the spine have no nerves or blood vessels. They're made of connective tissue, water, and fat. As we stand and sit during the day, the water is squeezed out of our disks by gravitational pressure and later slowly restored while we sleep. Because of this process, youngsters, whose bodies contain more water and less fat, are as much an inch taller when they wake up in the morning than they are at night. As we get older, the water content of our disks diminishes overall, reducing their individual thickness. This is one reason people get shorter with age. It's also one of the most common and severe causes of low back pain. (See the discussion of osteoarthritis in Chapter 9).

A substance like rice paper, called the annulus fibrosis, covers disks on the outside; inside they have a soft shiny center (the nucleus pulposis), which can be compared to a lichee nut. Spinal disks cushion the entire body, support the vertebral column, protect the nerves that exit the spine between the vertebral bones, and, as mentioned before, influence height. Pressure can deform and dehydrate the disks, but if the pressure isn't too great, they return to their original size and shape. Their flexibility gives them strength, but with limitations. Combine too strong an outside push or too hard a bump with restricted flexibility, and the bump picks up momentum, applying a magnified force and sometimes resulting in injury.

Many people want to know what happens when a disk slips. The answer is, if the outer wall (annulus fibrosis) of a disk is broken, its contents (nucleus pulposus) are often pushed into the hollow spaces within vertebral column, where nerves travel between the brain and every part of the body. The disk itself has no nerves and thus no feeling, but when it presses against a nerve, this irritates the nerves, which can cause great pain. Sometimes the discomfort is in the back, but more often pain occurs in the part of the body the nerve serves. (Much more about this is given in Chapter 9).

Doctor Joel Saal, associate director of research and education at the San Francisco Spine Institute in Daly City, California, has described the various flexible properties of the disk with accuracy and an eye to their actual dynamic function. This includes an ability to twist which is incompletely restrained by the tendons, ligaments, and the faceted joints themselves. Many physicians in the fields of orthopedics, rehabilitation, and neurology believe that overly forceful or violent twisting is more dangerous for disks than bending or tilting. There is still a great deal to learn, however, about the behavior of these delicate formations, which can be the cause of great difficulty.

If either ligaments or disks alone had to bear the pressures of movement, these structures would react to the stress by thickening over time or by shortening, which would restrict movement and change leverages, making them less useful to the individual. Obviously, working alone, either type of structure would be more liable to damage. But it is a shared burden by design. When you bend so much that the disk is in danger of breaking, then the ligament becomes taut, restraining further motion. If you try to bend even more, both the disk and the ligament present greater resistance. This cooperative effort improves leverage and safety, but when the body sustains abrupt, severe jolts, the disk can rupture (see Chapter 9).

Joints

The body has joints everywhere, from the big plateaus of the bending knees to the tiny articulated bones in the eardrums that communicate vibrations from the outside world. Joints are located at the junction of at least two bones and enable the bones to move in relation to each other. Like the spine, they have characteristics that both permit and confine movement.

The majority of joints in the spine have smooth, gleaming surfaces of cartilage. A rough capsule pleated like a curtain encloses each of these joints, which are bathed in a very slippery lubricating oil. Every vertebra has a joint at each of its four facets. When a joint bends to one side, the pleats unfold on the opposite side, holding in the lubricating fluid. When the joint is at rest, the covering folds along its pleats so that it doesn't take up a lot of room, disturb nearby structures, or become vulnerable to injury.

Two things commonly go wrong with the joints of the spine. The first is a problem with facet joints that commonly happens in young people. Imagine each vertebra as a short, fat person with two arms and two legs: the arms reach up to connect with the legs of the vertebra above, and the legs reach down to connect with the arms of the vertebra below. These tiny junctures are true joints; they have membranes, cartilage, and fluid—all the properties of any other joint in the body. Abrupt, heedless movement can make the facet joints slip out of their normal alignment. When this happens, the joints of one vertebra and the vertebra above or below it are no longer facing each other exactly but get locked in some other position. This is extremely painful, but chiropractic, massage, and physical therapy can realign the facets.

The second problem occurs in the elderly. Instead of a single event, it is the accumulation of many little traumas at the joint surface. Over time these injuries gradually produce permanent swellings and deformities on surfaces that worked best when they fit together perfectly. When the joint moves or supports weight, these irregularities bear all the pressure that is usually evenly distributed over its entire surface. These imperfections are osteoarthritis, a source of pain that is easy to reduce but impossible to cure.

Other Connective Tissue

The elements described so far—disks, tendons and ligaments are what anatomists call discrete structures. Other connective tissue is amorphous, but like those functional units I've described previously, it permits movement and enhances stability. Connective tissue is probably the most undervalued and least understood element in our backs. It begins just under the top layer of skin and is the warp and weft of the fabric of our bodies. As such, it supplies the general matrix in which all activity (including thought) takes place. Importantly, connective tissue is elastic in children; it becomes somewhat stringy and less resilient as we grow older.

What can go wrong with something so formless? Disorders of connective tissue include restrictive scarring, prolific fatty tissue, edema (swelling), and a variety of tumors, all of which may adversely affect the movements and structure of the spine. A scarred chest from a childhood burn may restrict reaching upward. This would cause you to overarch your back when stretching for something from an overhead kitchen cabinet. Lifting swollen legs to walk is more difficult than moving normal legs, and more likely to injure the sacroiliac joint. Some genetic connective tissue diseases can affect normal movement, causing back problems.

Modern manual medicine, an alternative treatment method that is now entering the mainstream of physical therapy, targets connective tissue to alleviate pain. One of its goals is to change the consistency and depth of attachment of connective tissue to the muscles and bones beneath it and to work toward a cure with stretching, compression, and "enforced" movement, using patients' own muscles to effect a therapeutic change.

Pain

Most back pain comes in two distinct varieties: musculoskeletal and neurological. When pain is musculoskeletal, at least one of the following hurts: muscles, ligaments, tendons, or joints. This kind of pain is generally gnawing, achy, and persistent. Picking up a heavy object the wrong way, repetitive actions like hitting a tennis ball, and structural malfunctions in the spine itself can cause this type of pain. If not reprovoked, it almost always disappears within 10 days. It rarely has serious consequences, but in the meantime it's very challenging to treat. Musculoskeletal pain accounts for two-thirds to three-quarters of all low back pain.

Neurological pain may originate in one place and be felt in another. The way nerve pain is communicated is sometimes compared to the way voices travel over telephone wires. If you were in New York speaking to someone in Los Angeles, and a wayward operator in Kansas City broke in on your call and yelled "help!," you would interpret the SOS as coming from California. Paradoxically, nerve pain may be caused by a problem with a disk, a structure that has no feeling. When an injured disk adds "noise" to the communication between spinal nerves serving the skin of the foot and your brain, your brain interprets that "noise" as a pain in the foot. In that case the pain is caused in one place but manifests in another. If pain in the back is accompanied by unpleasant sensations on or in the lower part of the body, including the legs, the likelihood is that you have a neurological problem.

Though you may have a pinched nerve in your back, sometimes you don't feel it there at all. The pain starts in the mid-buttock and seems to travel down the back of the leg. There may be a crackly or hypersensitive area on the surface of the skin, causing "buzzing," tingling, and hurting at the same time. You feel the pain two feet away from the place in the spine where the problem originates.

A third type of low back pain is really a combination of musculoskeletal and nerve pain. Most commonly, irritation of a nerve causes muscle spasm and temporary muscle pain. The inflammation of the nerve can come from many sources, from flu to direct trauma to muscular overuse. In the last situation, injury to the muscle causes blood and fluid to build up in the muscle. Swollen muscle tissue then presses against a nerve, disturbing its normal function. This is nerve pain that derives from a musculoskeletal source.

A jazz pianist and composer came to me this kind of combination problem. For many hours a day she was practicing the songs she intended to record for her first CD. And she was pushing herself further by feverishly working with a mouse while composing new music on her computer. When using the mouse this young woman had to move her arm in unfamiliar patterns that stressed her muscles. The muscles reacted by swelling. This caused pressure on her ulnar nerve, which controls almost all delicate finger movements.

Low back pain can result when overactivity makes buttock muscles swell; then these muscles can press on the sciatic nerve.

Pain Caused by Faulty Interactions

Faulty interaction among spinal elements is a great deal of the subject matter of this book. Faulty interactions cause some typically hard-to-diagnose kinds of back pain. If we consider all the mathematical combinations of the seven elements of the spine, the number of possibilities for the cause of a specific back pain begins at 5,040. Faulty interactions, because they take place only while a person is standing or moving, are extremely difficult for a physician to pinpoint. A doctor might see a vertebra out of place on an X ray or MRI (magnetic resonance image). However, the image doesn't show changes that occur between the vertebra and the nerve when their owner is in motion, so it's impossible to be certain the pain-causing problem isn't in the buttock nine inches away.

BETWEEN VERTEBRAE AND DISKS

One type of faulty interaction between two vertebrae and their disks is called spondylolisthesis (see Chapter 9). The forward slippage of one vertebra causes misalignment of the entire spinal column above it, producing stress and strain in the person trying to balance. Think of a waiter trying to control a stack of plates, one of which is sliding out of the pile. Add to the unbalanced spinal stack the movements of legs, arms, and head. The demands on the muscles of the lower back to hold the structure vertical can cause painful fatigue and spasm.

MRIs may show that one vertebra has slid a few millimeters beyond its usual placement on the vertebrae below it, but physicians still usually read these imaging reports as "essentially normal." If the patient complains of constant and severe pain in the muscles beside the spine and in the buttock and hip, and the doctor might prescribe a nonsteroidal painkiller that doesn't help.

The slippage may not press on any nerves in the neural canal behind the vertebra, and it might not threaten disk rupture or push the vertebra totally off the one that supports it from below. Nevertheless, this microscopic misalignment is still a cause of spinal instability that disrupts the symmetry and balance of the body, greatly adding to the burden of adjustment for a large and changing group of muscles. A small slippage of the vertebra can compel one muscle to tighten and work harder than its counterparts above, below, or opposite. Not surprisingly, intense muscular pain is produced in various parts of the back and may be associated with severe pain in the buttock as well as in the lumbar spine.

Between Disks and Nerves

Faulty interaction between disks and nerves is a common, major cause of low back pain that will be discussed throughout this book. The faulty interaction occurs when a disk collapses and the material of which it is made presses against a nerve. Small fragments of the disk stimulate the nerve to feel pain, but often not at the site of its original cause. A disk-and-nerve problem occurring in the L4-L5 vertebral segment can press the nerve that exits at L5-S1 (that is, between the fifth lumbar and the first sacral vertebrae); this produces burning along the outside of the calf and on the skin between the first two toes. A patient experiencing pain like this may mistakenly think he or she needs a podiatrist. Surgery is often successfully performed to correct this structurally based faulty interaction.

In the Joint between Two Bones

The change in position of a sacroiliac joint while shoveling snow, for example, is the precursor of pain caused by a faulty interaction in the joint between two bones. The person naturally gravitates away from the discomfort caused by an initial injury, shifting the weight away from that side. But the leg on the affected side still has to move. As a result, the muscles of the lumbar spine on the affected side become so tight they cause a spasm. The spasm affects the muscles over time, and can actually cause extreme, long-lasting, and hard-to-cure pain that appears much farther up in the cervical spine, or even as headaches. The problem lies in that sacroiliac joint, but the pain is felt in the neck or head because the balancing act that muscles must perform results in changes of posture, carriage, and muscle tone.

AMONG LIGAMENTS, TENDONS, AND OTHER
CONNECTIVE TISSUE

The following scenario provides an example of pain caused by faulty interactions among ligaments, tendons, and connective tissue. A right-handed father throws a baseball to his son, pulls a ligament on the left side of his spine, and strains the muscle between two ribs. This stays inflamed and sore for quite some time. As a result of favoring the injured side, there is chronic stretching of the connective tissue on the right side. The man sways slightly to the left when he walks. Within weeks, the asymmetry in his gait has become habitual. Now, in addition to the original injury, the gait abnormality is causing a problem in the hip. Because of the small incessant impacts of walking, discomfort is spreading both downward to the knee and upward to the spine.

Putting It All Together

The living spine harmonizes movements of the arms and legs with bones cushioned and connected by shock-absorbing, flexible disks and joints. It allows not only for symmetrical movements (in which the left and right sides of the body are balanced), such as typing at a keyboard, but also gives us a scaffold for accomplishing asymmetrical tasks like painting a picture or winding twine into a ball. The nerves—which course through the spinal canal longitudinally—exit between the vertebrae, and branch throughout the body. They have two functions. They direct muscular activity and receive feedback about objects and reports on whether distances, weights, and velocities have been properly estimated. Connective tissue protects and adjusts the entire package by passively resisting extreme changes of position. The spine can be seen as the centerpiece of the body. Our spines are rigid enough to oppose the downward tug of gravity and help us remain upright, but they're also adjustable enough to allow us innumerable combinations of balanced movement.

Our spines are paradoxical—firm but flexible, strong but fragile. Until something goes wrong, it's easy to take one's spine for granted. An awareness and appreciation of the spine's complexity—during movement, while supporting us, or at rest—should inspire us to use it carefully.

CHAPTER 2

Diagnosis

THE BASIS OF CURE

Often a patient's opening remark to me is, "I came to you because I don't want surgery."

Worry is a natural part of not feeling up to par, but when it comes to low back pain, there's little cause for alarm. Less than 1 percent of my patients with backache need to go under the knife, and there's an extremely high success rate for those who do choose corrective surgery.

Many people who come to me for help, however, are at the other end of the spectrum. Far from fearing the worst, they're in my office just trying to confirm their suspicion that they need a doctor, or investigating how to choose the right one (see Chapter 3).

No matter how they might be categorized, I've observed over and over again that patients generally know more about their own condition than they themselves or their doctors give them credit for. Some genuine listening by the physician often shows that the person who's feeling the pain has an intuition about its seriousness and constructive ideas for its cure.

For any patient who needs attention from a clinician, entering the

---

---

medical system can be daunting. It's a labyrinth, shrouded in rumor and novelty, with shifting areas of focus and control, Greco-Roman labels, and baffling technological refinements.

Though the system is complex and confusing, the patient who experiences pain for a significant length of time has little choice but to participate in it. Then his or her role becomes crucial. I firmly believe the person whose back is aching must become partners with the physician during the analytical, creative process of making a diagnosis. After the correct diagnosis has been attained, the patient must participate in making treatment plans and should carry those plans out conscientiously.

Years of experience have taught me that patients who are also educated citizens, ready and willing to work with their doctors, have a significantly better chance of finding the cause of their back pain, of mastering that pain, and then achieving a permanent cure.

If this book is to be of any use to you, the first principle it should communicate is that most of the time you need information about what's wrong before anything much can be done about it. Obviously a condition or disease of unknown origins is more difficult to deal with than one whose cause has been found, and it usually takes the right specialist to identify the cause. But, you ask, doesn't that make the problem a frustrating catch 22? Doesn't that mean you need a diagnosis before you can decide whom to ask to make a diagnosis?

Not exactly. Your hunches about your condition may be correct. At least, you have nothing more to go on before seeking medical help. If you just took a nasty backward fall and now you have a sharp pain in that part of your spine each time you stand, then hurry to an orthopedist, who will likely request imaging studies. If you were pulling the canoe paddle through the water when a sharp pain started in your own "stern," an appointment with an osteopath would be a logical first step. Chapter 3 describes the various specialties and suggests how to decide when a doctor's appointment is necessary; Chapter 9 outlines how your pain can guide you to the proper healer.

Before You See the Doctor

No matter which physician you decide to see first, two factors will be used to make a diagnosis: the medical history and the physical exam. Familiarizing yourself with the major aspects of each will prepare you to make the best use of them. Before you go to a doctor, it's in your own best interest to ask yourself basic questions about your condition and to have the answers to those questions ready. These answers to your own queries about symptoms and possible causes are often sufficient to narrow the choice of who would be the logical person to perform the initial exam. The thought you've already given to your own problem will help you make most efficient use of your time when you do see the doctor. If you've tried a specialist and haven't solved your problem, the question-and-answer self-examination will aid you in making a choice about which specialist to try next.

It's often helpful to think about and describe your pain using the third person ("he felt," "she feels" rather than "I felt") before seeing the doctor. A pen and small pad of paper are invaluable tools for jotting down symptoms and listing questions to ask the doctor, and then for noting the answers to those questions, so that later at home you can review exactly what the doctor told you.

Look for patterns in the pain you feel, look for variations, and write it all down. Edit that information to make better use of your time with the doctor. Include not only a description of *what* you feel but *when* you feel it, including the time of day, activity, position, situation, relation to mealtime, and seemingly irrelevant factors, like weather and wardrobe, especially shoes.

A common problem patients face in the doctor's office is not being able to locate the exact spot of the pain. It's not difficult, once you're there on the examining table, to avoid the feeling that you've flunked a test. Just as you once studied your spelling words before the weekly quiz in school, you can practice in advance for the doctor's exam. Think about what movements and positions cause your pain, and try to reproduce it at home. Lean against the furniture, if you need to, or get a friend to help. The visit with the doctor *can* seem a little like a test in school, but this time the way to get an A is to figure out what's wrong.

If you're lucky enough to find what makes you feel better—for instance, sleeping on the hard floor rather than on your soft bed—you might be able to cancel your doctor's appointment. That's what happened to a journalist we'll call Kathryn. She did some fanny walks in her exercise class at the YWCA. Shortly after one particularly strenuous session, she experienced severe low back pain. She says it was dumb luck that made her lie on her bed in a fetal position, but actually she intuitively stumbled onto her own cure.

For those who can't cure themselves using simple, safe techniques such as over-the-counter painkillers, ice, two or three days of bed rest, and a few weeks of cautious living, a visit to a physician is advisable.

Taking the Medical History

Doctors almost always begin their investigation into the cause of the symptoms by taking a medical history. Much more than a list of childhood diseases, of medications you've taken, of other physicians you've seen, the history consists of a rich description not only of what's wrong, but of your activities, your inherited characteristics, even your emotions. Medical schools teach that nine out of 10 factors in a diagnosis come from the patient's medical history. Sometimes what's wrong becomes immediately obvious during the interview, sometimes it's difficult to ferret out, but most of the time the physical exam just confirms the educated guess the physician (and often the patient) has already made.

D I D   Y O U   K N O W ?

Recently, a group of patients filled out questionnaires about their histories and then went to the doctor. Doctors agreed with 77 percent of patients' classification of themselves as fit for work and with 90 percent of those who felt they couldn't work.

Help with techniques for answering many of the questions the doctor will ask during the taking of the medical history (how to describe the character of the pain, for example) is given in the chapters on symptoms. Reading these chapters will sharpen your descriptive skills. Your aim when describing your problem to the doctor is to be as specific and concise as possible—to choose your words with such care that they will illuminate your condition for the clinician. Bear in mind, when you're sitting across the desk discussing your history with your doctor, that this is the moment when you're most likely to present the information that will lead to your cure.

PREVIOUS AND CURRENT SYMPTOMS

All medical histories of low back pain should give full details about when you first felt the pain and any possibly related events or repetitive activity in the few days before the pain began. Often there is noth-

---

D I D   Y O U   K N O W ?

Statistics show your employment status, what tasks you perform at work, your smoking and drinking habits, previous treatments, and your general state of mind can influence what you tell your doctor about your symptoms, and can also have an effect on the type of treatment the doctor recommends.

---

ing—no fall, for example, or memory of lifting something unusually heavy—that the patient can pinpoint. Still, the examining physician can learn a great deal from hearing what happened during the minutes, hours, or first few days after the pain started. Did it radiate? Was it associated with feelings like electric shocks? Were there strange sensations of tingling, pins-and-needles, or cold? (See Chapter 7.) If so, where? If there was numbness or weakness, where was it? (See Chapters 6 and 8.) Does anything—for example, changing position or lying down—make the pain better? What, if anything—sex, driving, lifting heavy objects, going up or down a hill or stairs, or exercise—makes the pain worse?

Like someone studying the origins of a conflict that has escalated slowly until it developed into war, the physician will attempt to understand the dynamics of your problem. Has anything changed since the pain began? Is it getting better, worse, or staying the same? Has the pain itself altered, going from sharp, for example, to a throbbing ache?

It's important to tell your physician about any major change in your normal routine. For some people, the original symptoms cause a change in behavior that makes everything worse. A classic case of this is the overweight museum official who had to stop exercising because of back pain. Almost immediately his stomach muscles lost tone. This made him subject to extra muscle fatigue, which caused more discomfort in his back and sacroiliac joints. Another typical example is the woman who began hunching her shoulders to change her center of gravity and relieve the pain in her back. Changes in posture often cause new problems, and in this case those changes made her neck hurt many times more than her lower back.

A physician doing a complete history will ask you about your diet, recent acquisitions like new chairs and cars, menstruation, and past surgeries. Backache associated with other aches and pains, perhaps in your head or mid-thigh, can help diagnose generalized conditions that could be serious, like multiple sclerosis or diabetes.

If you have previously experienced the sort of pain you have now, the doctor will need the details, including how the earlier situation was resolved. Fever, night sweats, a history of tuberculosis, a weight

---

SELF-EXAMINATION

Discrepancy in the length of your legs can contribute to back pain. You can test for this yourself and report the results to your doctor during the physical exam. Sit at the edge of a hard-bottomed flat chair (a slanted seat won't give correct results). With your shoes off, place your feet side by side and flat on the floor. Your legs should be straight from knees to ankles. Using a mirror, or with the help of a friend, look at your knees. Are your kneecaps parallel? If not, an eighth-inch discrepancy is normal, ⅜ inch borders on significant, and ¼ inch is enough to cause pain and need correction.

---

loss or gain, swelling, problems in the arm and leg joints, and a history of back problems in the family may also be significant.

PRESENTING THE INFORMATION

The purpose of the medical history is to help make a diagnosis and effect a cure, but it doesn't work that way for everyone. For some patients a definitive diagnosis is like the proverbial pot of gold at the end of the rainbow—always in sight but just out of reach. If you are one of the thousands who has gone from doctor to doctor unsuccessfully seeking a cure, the first question to ask yourself is, Why have the doctors been led astray? Could it be that you are unwittingly concealing crucial information during the taking of the history? Rather than presenting the facts evenly, do you have a diagnosis you are favoring? Are you excluding some facts in order to convince the doctor? For example, are you afraid to admit how bad it is?

Report Difficult Information First   A singer friend of mine helped solve her romantic difficulties by making it a habit to begin each session with her psychotherapist with what she *least* wanted to report.

The same technique—starting with the information most difficult to confide—could help you give your history. For example, one patient recovering from a slipped disk was embarrassed to tell me she had ignored my advice and used the rowing machine at her gym. Yet once I knew this crucial fact I could direct her physical therapist to help her with arching exercises and hands-on techniques, including massage.

Get the Facts Straight Think hard to be sure you're stating the facts correctly. A man came to me in December. "Apparently I'm allergic to October," he said. "My back hurts and my fingers always get numb only during that month. But this year it didn't go away." He was mistaken: he was diagnosed with a connective tissue disease that narrowed his spine. Limited range of motion required him to bend over farther and use his wrists more each year. That led to inflamed carpal tunnels (compression of the median nerve, which controls the thumb) after raking fall leaves. It also gave him chronic low back pain. When he reflected on all this, he remembered the pain had also lasted for months the year before.

Try not to "argue" your case to convince the doctor to agree with your own preconceived diagnosis, leaving out or forgetting important facts that might lead in other directions. As I said before, you may very well have the best first impression of what your problem is, but if that fails, your doctor needs your assistance in careful analysis and detective work.

Avoid Exaggeration and Minimizing Don't exaggerate or minimize your pain. Without meaning to, some patients actually deny or overestimate the reason for visiting the doctor in order to prove a point. What you're trying to prove may be an honest misapprehension, a way to score a victory in a domestic quarrel, a response to something that happened with another doctor, or it may actually be correct. Just remember that the way you make your point influences the choices the examining practitioner makes about how to proceed.

A demanding patient who once visited me was certain she had a "pinched nerve." When I read over five reports from other doctors, it was clear from the tests they had performed and the medicines they'd tried that none of them had believed her. I had an inkling that was because when she described her symptoms she made many asides about her dissatisfaction not only with members of the medical profession but with family members and even friends she accused of not having enough sympathy for what she was going through.

I tried testing her for what she thought was wrong and found to my surprise that she had been right: she did actually have an entrapped nerve. When I began treating her for that, she found relief and underwent a blessed personality change.

Some people minimize their pain as a way of reducing their own anxiety about it and about the frightening idea that it might never go away. After I was quoted in a newspaper article, a number of people called me. I was so impressed with the chronicity and severity of their pain that I opened the office on Sundays. One Sunday morning my assistant and I looked out the window to see two black stretch limousines pull up. Several men emerged from one car, looked around, then fanned out along our part of the block, apparently keeping watch, we didn't know why. Then a serious-looking man dressed in a sharkskin suit whose jacket bulged on the left side emerged from the other car and held the door open for the man—a tall, pleasant-looking fellow with a bright, short-sleeved sports shirt—who was obviously the patient.

These two men, who could have stepped right out of *The Godfather,* appeared in my office a few minutes later. "Happy," the man in the sports shirt, told me he had been in pain for seven years, had sought treatment only on Wednesdays and Fridays when he was in Queens, and only from a Transcendental Meditator, whose word he took as gospel.

"Where does it bother you," I asked.

His companion jumped up, stuck his mug in mine and declared belligerently, "The boss is fine. Nothing bothers him. You get it? Nothing!"

"It's not so bad," Happy answered stoically.

In this case an employee was inappropriately defending his boss, and both were minimizing the severe pain "Happy" was suffering. Many patients don't realize they're inappropriately acting as their own "bodyguards." Minimizing can take the form of repeating a non-threatening test or repeatedly seeing a "friendly" doctor, instead of entertaining more difficult tactics, such as seeing a specialist or losing those extra 25 pounds, either of which might actually cure chronic pain.

Avoid Confusing Language While some patients defend themselves by overstating or denying what's wrong, others confuse themselves and their clinicians by describing their problems in detail so overly minute it is difficult to recognize as real human experience. A man once described his pain as "staccato miniburst of subthreshold agony."

That sounded objective, it sounded important, but it made me scratch my head. And eventually it led to a question: if these minibursts were subthreshold, how was he able to feel them? The agony, he replied, was that he couldn't exactly feel those bursts of agony, and had a lot of trouble describing them. Methodical questioning revealed a strange sensation that came and went and seemed to the patient to be too mundane to actually be true. Sometimes for minutes, but usually for seconds, the skin on this man's legs felt as if it were stretched to the breaking point. He showed me the sensitive area, precisely outlining the region served by the L5 nerve root. There were telltale signs of herpes, too. One medicine and four weeks later his pain had disappeared.

Use Medical Terms Accurately Some patients try successfully to catch the doctor's attention by using medical red flags. When describing the character of their pain, for instance, they use words like "exquisite" (severe, commanding attention) or "lancinating" (knife-like). That's fine. Just be sure to use the right term. Though you may not be able to cure yourself, it makes sense to learn the vocabulary of what ails you, including the terminology of physiology, anatomy, and pathology. The more educated you are, the more active a role you can play in your own cure.

Participate Actively in the Diagnosis Having failed to receive help in the past, some patients develop a negative attitude they apply to the present, inadvertently standing in the way of each new opportunity to achieve a diagnosis and cure. Previous failures discourage these people to the point where they relinquish responsibility. I've seen patients who, when questioned either directly or indirectly, will say: "Well, you're the doctor, you tell *me* where it hurts."

One of those patients, a stockbroker in her forties, came to me recently after spending a month at a well-known diagnostic center. "I've had every orifice under siege for so long my family has nick-named me 'Sarajevo'," she laughed bitterly. "But I still have absolutely no idea what's wrong with me."

Checking into the center was a surrender, an admission of the degree that this woman's illness was changing her life. But once she was in the hands of clinicians there, she unquestioningly knuckled under to the "authority" of the specialists. "I let them do whatever they wanted," she actually told me. "After all, they're the experts." That passivity had contributed to the failure of her mission to cure herself.

It was a shame she didn't know how important it is to encourage clinicians, even world-renowned specialists, to make sure they have the answers to questions every medical history should contain: Has the cause of the pain been found? If so, how can it be treated? If not, how can the possible problems be narrowed down until a conclusive diagnosis can be reached? What are the likeliest causes of the problem?

Use Communication Aids Where Necessary Accurate communication is essential to giving and receiving a medical history. If you are in a foreign land or the doctor is from one, I advise bringing a translator along. Hearing aids should not be left at home. One patient told me he'd remembered his earpiece, then said, "But when I realized I was going to see a *doctor*, I was sure I'd be understood." Yes, but communication didn't go the other way. The patient didn't understand detailed questions I asked, the answers to which were critical to his diagnosis and proper referral. Luckily his daughter was reachable by phone.

WORKING WITH YOUR DOCTOR

Don't regard the taking of your medical history as a hostile cross-examination on the witness stand. It has been my experience that the patients most likely to leave my office feeling better are those who treat the initial history as a conversation. They may have an opinion about what's wrong with them, or they may have come up with a blank. Either way, they're flexible and willing to entertain new ideas.

Complaints about the past don't belong in the medical history. Telling the current physician the qualifications, office manner, and other particulars of physicians who have failed you is not constructive for you or your current doctor. These failures should be considered mutual. If you are a patient who has had chronic pain and you have gone from doctor to doctor, tests and treatment alternatives have already been attempted. If these tests haven't come up with conclusions, you should demand the historical investigation and intensive physical exam given by physiatrists (specialists in physical medicine and rehabilitation). Remember that discovering what you *don't* have might be easier than identifying what actually is wrong, and may be a helpful way to start. Patience is necessary to eliminate, one by one, the finite number of possibilities in order to focus attention on the likely options, and finally arrive at an answer.

Your ability to analyze yourself and your behavior with honesty can help the experts cure you. Unbelievable as it seems, I have seen a number of highly skilled professionals whose pain appears to give them a strange type of comfort and satisfaction. Their mind-set reminds me of the story of the mermaid who fell in love with the sailor, but could only dance beautifully as long as she felt the pain of dancing on knives.

An example is a highly successful stockbroker who spent long hours seated, gazing at, and responding to what transpired on her computer screen. At the close of business, she often rose and said, "My God, I've been in pain all day." Worse, occasionally she could not rise from her chair at all. Early on I suggested she could help herself by placing the monitor and the keyboard higher up so she could stand while working. No, she said, that wouldn't be convenient. Then I came up with another idea. She could have two monitors—one high, one low—so she could alter her position from time to time. She resisted everything. "Oh, it's not really *so* bad," she told me every time I found a possible solution. I began to understand that underneath she felt as long as something was wrong, everything was all right.

Another member of the financial world, this time a commodities broker, was a textbook case of how competing with the doctor can stand in the way of good medical treatment. This gentleman flew in from out of state to see me, and almost from the beginning of our meeting, he signaled that he had a type A personality. Though he seemed to need to impress me by telling me stories of plans to consummate big deals and even by calling attention to his tan, at first we got along very well.

Then, as I was taking his history, he noticed my watch. "Does that watch have a timer?" he asked me. When told that it did, he eagerly suggested that I trade mine for his, though the timepiece adorning his wrist cost at least ten times more than my plastic digital model, a fact I felt it necessary to point out while refusing his offer.

In our subsequent interactions this man asked me personal questions about my finances, always implying the obvious—that he had more money than I. He made a number of other attempts to "best" me. I don't know why he initiated this contest, but his need to compete with me made it much more difficult to figure out that his pain came from jogging, and to get him to use the proper orthotic (shoe insert).

Instead of working against me, some patients really believe the old adage that two heads are better than one. A quick-minded, able lobbyist with chronic pain came to see me from the West Coast and told me there were four men in his group who were under rather extreme strain. Of the four, one had had heart attacks, one had had strokes, one had metastatic cancer. "Then there's me," he said. "Nobody in my neck of the woods can find out what I've got."

After an hour-and-a-half exam, I told him that I thought he had piriformis syndrome—a situation in which the piriformis muscle in the buttock presses on the sciatic nerve resulting in severe pain while sitting but a normal MRI. I assured him that physical therapy could provide a cure. I wrote him an elaborate prescription and offered to confer by phone with a physical therapist he would find when he returned home. He laughed and asked for the name of a nearby hotel. "If no one out there could diagnose me," he said, "how much luck do you think they'd have with the treatment?" I was amazed at his approach, but I agreed to oversee his treatment until he felt better. It took a week.

Like the needle in the haystack, diagnosis may be hard to find, but once in hand, almost everyone will know how to proceed. Unfortunately the knowledge doesn't always inspire a patient to put himself out. I have seen more than one patient who has lived in misery for fifteen years, yet refused to travel an hour twice a week for two months in order to achieve a complete cure.

A patient's closed mind can prevent the doctor from taking even the first steps toward a cure. One pugnacious man of European origin, whom I'll call Ivan, blustered as he returned to my office without any appointment. "You don't do things right," he shouted. "You don't do things like the other doctors" (who had failed to help him).

I tried to explain.

"I can't hear you!" he shouted louder.

Everyone's attention was riveted on us. Finally, raising my voice as high as his, I exclaimed, "We know what's wrong with you, we think we can help you!"

There was a pause. Then, in a stage whisper he replied, "I know. Why are you shouting?"

"I thought you couldn't hear me."

He dryly stated, "I hear what I want to hear," and left.

Ivan literally slammed the door on a partnership between us. Another patient made the mistake of letting a long-standing friendship come between her and help. She broke the rule that loyalty to a doctor should be based completely on the quality of the care received and nothing else. A "personage" in the New York art and theater world, this eighty-five-year-old woman had gone to the same doctor for so long that the two of them had grown old together. The physician should have retired decades before. He could no longer give a basic exam, let alone diagnose the problems with this sweet woman's hip joint. But the woman didn't feel she could withdraw her patronage without hurting her old buddy. Finally her son convinced her to keep her original physician as a friend and to find a new one to provide medical care. The story has a happy ending. Her hip was replaced under local anesthesia. I saw her on a TV talk show a month ago.

Be bold when necessary. Tom, a computer specialist from California's Silicon Valley, had terrible, intractable low back pain for seven years. In spite of his problem, he had managed to find a girlfriend, propose, and then get married. About a year later his physical condition began to cause problems in his relationship with his wife. Because he was an intelligent fellow who worked with computers, he had researched back pain thoroughly. He had read the articles and taken their advice; he had gone to specialists and superspecialists.

This poor person sat and told me his whole story, but with interruptions. Several times he excused himself and went out of the room. Finally I asked him for an explanation. It seems that in addition to terrible back pain, there was an intestinal problem. He'd had intermittent diarrhea he attributed to stress caused by the pain. I sent him for a simple blood test. It came back with elevated levels of eosinophils (a kind of blood cell). That prompted stool analysis. This man had somehow caught parasites—to be exact, dog hookworm—and had been their victim for seven long years!

Chronic pain had had an effect on Tom's posture, which needed correction with physical therapy, and the longtime roomers and boarders in his body needed eviction. Together we worked out a complete treatment plan to be carried out in California. I followed Tom for about six weeks by telephone, and when I spoke to him last he was planning a second honeymoon.

The Physical Exam

What happened with Tom is an example of how the giving and taking of the history must end with the doctor observing the patient directly. A physician might have an idea about a diagnosis, but there's more to diagnosing than meets the ear. To be absolutely sure, eyes must be used to look for swelling, asymmetries, withering, rash, and other symptoms, and hands must be laid on to test muscle strength, to examine skin sensitivity, to physically find the problem, or to decide on diagnostic tests.

During the physical exam, you as the patient are both active (moving voluntarily) and passive (letting the doctor do the moving for you). Because it's so important for the doctor to be able to look at and touch you, it's necessary to get undressed. Your job is not only to cooperate with all tests, but to be sure the physician feels the painful place. It's helpful to show the doctor any maneuvers and pressures that cause pain, make existing pain worse, or relieve it.

Not being able to find the painful place often happens because changes in position make muscles slide over each other and obscure the trouble spot. The obscuring muscles are resilient, so that pushing on them in search of the painful location is like pressing on several cushions. You will avoid this problem, and the worry that you've wasted an important part of your time with the doctor, by locating the pain to the best of your ability *before* you leave home for the doctor's office.

Standard Beginnings

Range of Motion   Range of motion is one of the first things that's checked if a patient complains of back pain. If the pelvis, legs, and back move properly, you should be asked to do standing and seated forward bends. A watchful, discerning doctor is alert to the possibility that your legs are of different lengths, that your lumbar vertebrae don't move properly, or that your sacrum is unbalanced as it slides within its iliac joints.

Muscle Strength   Simple tests of muscle strength are next on the list. You will be asked to push with all your might against the doctor's hand, to pull, and to squeeze. You will walk on heels and tiptoes.

You may have weakness that is gross or subtle, and it may be symmetrical or asymmetrical (the same or different on each side of your body). Whatever its nature, weakness is almost always relevant. Weakness may cause back pain, or it may be the effect of back pain (see Chapter 8). If you're weak somewhere, make sure the examining physician is aware of it.

Sensation   Changes in sensation also work both ways—they can either cause low back pain or be the result of it. Numbness alters the way you walk, climb stairs, and sit, all of which may cause low back pain. On the other hand, a pinched nerve can cause low back pain and reduce muscle strength and sensation. The most common test for problems with sensation involves light pinpricks to map out affected skin areas (see Chapter 7).

Reflexes   Testing of reflexes is fundamental to a physical exam. Reflexes involve a sensory nerve and a motor nerve. When stimulated, the sensory nerve activates the motor nerve in the spinal cord. This transmits a signal to the muscle, causing it to contract—for example, your leg jerks when your knee is struck with a reflex hammer. Since reflexes occur at the spinal-cord level, you can't control them voluntarily. If the muscles, nerves, and sensory apparatus are normal, then reflexes will reflect this. The doctor's little hammer is used not only on the front of the knee but the front and back of the ankles and bottom of the foot as well. Different reflexes give information about the spinal cord at different levels.

Reflex testing should not only note lost reflexes, but also discover abnormally brisk ones. An overreaction can escalate until it produces spasticity (a condition such as cerebral palsy that makes muscles contract involuntarily).

Spasm   A spasm occurs when the muscle contracts and remains tightly contracted for a period of time, without voluntary control. The experienced physician can feel the enlarged, tightened muscles in spasm. Muscles in spasm are working, and the exertion causes them to grow. Let me explain. The bodies of all humans and animals have an engineering defect: When muscles contract, they need more blood, but in reality continued contraction closes the capillaries (tiny blood vessels) and reduces blood flow to the muscles just when they need it most. The lack of blood during spasm causes severe pain that is often grossly underrated by doctors.

Spasm is often quickly and permanently cured by simple stretching. I know this because of my own experience of having surgery on my shoulder. Afterward, while lying in my hospital bed the pain made me press the button on the morphine pump I was attached to with terrible frequency. At first I resisted my doctor's suggestion that I have physical therapy right then and there to stretch the painful muscle, thinking this pain must be too severe for mere spasm, but I gave in when he insisted. A physical therapist arrived at my bedside, and after working with me for five minutes, my pain disappeared forever.

Pulses   In a thorough exam a physician feels for pulses in blood flow at the inside of the ankle, the top of the foot, the front of the ankle, behind the knee, and at both groins. If one or more of these are abnormal, other pulses, even in the abdomen, must be checked. Chronic low back pain can have vascular origins (reflecting defects in the arteries). This is uncommon but serious, and needs to be looked for and ruled out.

Balance and Coordination   By simply standing with your eyes closed, remaining erect even when the doctor pushes you gently, and standing on one foot, the doctor can measure your equilibrium. Poor balance may prompt "guarding" responses in which muscles tire from overwork. If you have been experiencing loss of balance, even without actually falling, this could have caused sprain, strain, and joint derangements (minor displacents) anywhere, from your neck to toes.

Coordination is next. You should be asked to slide one heel from your opposite knee down the shin to the ankle. Then the doctor will observe you sitting, getting up from your chair, standing, and even lying down. If you are not watched going from a sitting to a standing position, the physician is missing something important; because everyone performs this action many times a day, any abnormality may precipitate back pain. It often shows problems such as poor management of your body's center of gravity (forward tilting of the torso shifts your weight and strains your back), leg weakness (which causes clumsy movement that can injure your lower back), and poor range of motion at the hip (which prompts overarching of the back). This simple test can also turn up a condition called dysmetria, which is the inability to move a body part to a designated place intentionally.

Poor coordination of gross movements (like raising the thigh) with fine movements (like supporting your weight "ballerina style" on the toes of one foot) can cause lumbar and thoracic back pain. Poor judgment of short distances can make merely getting up challenging and stressful.

Tests of coordination with alternating movements such as walking or bringing the forefingers together with arms out straight in front of you, and tests for balance, which is controlled by the central nervous system, may reveal an exact location in the brain that directly or indirectly causes low back pain. Possibly because of educational differences in past decades, or because of physical dissimilarities, men generally use their hips to maintain and regain balance, while women use their ankles.

Though balance has its own center in the brain, other factors, including poor coordination, weakness, numbness or joint problems at the hips, knees or ankles can make you unsteady on your feet. These possibilities should be explored.

Gait   Your doctor should watch you take a short walk back and forth in the examining room. When a person walks normally, all the joints and muscles work in efficient coordination with the center of gravity, which is generally the point halfway between the navel and genitals, an inch or two in front of the sacrum. Gait abnormalities that a trained expert observes during an office visit can point to numerous important causes of back pain.

Fear (after a stroke, for example), weakness, or a shorter leg may cause some people to take a longer step with one leg than with the other. This causes pain, usually on the side of the shorter step and often halfway between the spine and that hip (quadratus lumborum, the muscle connecting your lowest ribs with the back rim of the pelvis). When the cause is found and remediated, the back pain caused by this gait abnormality disappears.

Another example of a gait abnormality causing back pain is a common one. For many reasons (knee pain, a sliver, ill-fitting shoes, a charlie horse, etc.), people favor one leg (limp) when walking. This should be easy to spot, but is often hard to correct. If your pain increases with walking, you're probably in for some gait-training sessions with a physical therapist.

Dysfunctional feet (for example, when the big toe has insufficient range of motion) can cause pain in the hip that radiates to the groin, or pain in the knee, in the sacroiliac joints, or broadly across the lower back. To make matters worse, upper back and neck pain can accompany these other aches after periods of walking.

If your hip hurts or gives out during walking, or if back pain increases with standing or walking, try to show your doctor *where* in the gait cycle this occurs. Is it when your foot leaves the ground, when it comes forward, when the heel hits the ground, or when your foot is bearing weight? Is it when the toe is pushing off at the beginning of the next step? Gait is often underexamined by doctors, and you should be sure it isn't neglected during your physical exam.

Unusual Symptoms

During a physical exam, in addition to showing the doctor to the best of your ability just exactly where it hurts, make sure the physician looks at anything you think is unusual. In a strange case a seemingly unrelated problem turned out to be the answer. Susan, an athletic fifteen-year-old high school sophomore, woke up one morning and found her backache had turned into something much worse: she couldn't walk. Her parents brought her to me. We looked at everything—did MRIs, EMGs, and extensive blood work—and found nothing but an eye infection. That seemingly unimportant infection turned out to be the key. Eventually a sophisticated way of measuring nerve conduction velocity within the spinal column (SSEP) showed some-

thing related to the teenager's recent growth spurt. Her bones, growing faster than her nerves, had pulled her spinal cord down and exerted pressure on her whole nervous system, right up to and including
her optic nerve, prompting the eye infection. Once we knew what was
wrong, we gave her physical therapy and taught her some adaptations. Now, two years later, she's playing basketball on her high school
team.

Diagnostic Tests

Unless there's a clear reason to suspect a specific diagnosis that can
be turned up only by expensive tests like MRIs and CT scans, these
tests (described in Chapter 11) should not be done. Ask the doctor for
an explanation and reasons for prescribing or requesting these types
of diagnostic studies. Also ask which test results change treatment.
How likely are they?

Responding to Your Diagnosis

The happiest conclusion of a visit to the doctor is the news that your
problem has a name, that it's not serious, and that it can be easily
treated and / or will cure itself. I find this happens in the vast majority of cases. In a normal, thorough office visit of an hour and a half,

it's possible to categorize and begin to treat the problems of as many as 90 percent of the patients who come to me with low back pain, and to prescribe treatment.

There are times, however, when a diagnosis isn't definitive. The physician may be somewhat unsure or even mistaken. If you are given a diagnosis, it is perfectly reasonable for you to inquire how certain that diagnosis is, what ought to happen next, and what that will involve.

Of course, you might fall into that small group of patients whose diagnosis is elusive. A good doctor is capable of saying "I don't know," and that honesty indicates a mind still open to inquiry. If at the end of the examination you have no firm diagnosis, you should ask what the possibilities are. Then you and your doctor should discuss the next step in finding a diagnosis and work together to uncover the best avenue of investigation—diagnostic tests, another physician, a trial of therapy, or an adjustment of daily routine.

While usually welcome because of the promise of cure, a diagnosis can at other times be displeasing or frightening. A few patients have trouble accepting a diagnosis when it's given. They've mesmerized themselves into looking for an aesthetically pleasing or morally satisfying explanation for their prolonged and seemingly undeserved pain. Occasionally I see a patient who feels guilty enough to discard an explanation unless it contains a fault or action for which the person can take blame. My advice is that, no matter how unacceptable the diagnosis sounds, at least give it a chance before rejecting it. If it's something like, "You really should give up running," my advice is to see how close to this activity you can come. For example, can you ride a bicycle? How can you know if and when you can run again?

For a frightening diagnosis like multiple sclerosis (MS), you will need your wits about you. First, since emotions can cloud memory, write down the name of your condition. Ask your physician how likely it is that you really have it. Find out the best and worst you can expect, given your diagnosis. Then plan your first step for coping, for example, filling a prescription, getting further diagnostic testing, or getting a second opinion.

Remember, your diagnosis is different from your symptoms. The diagnosis identifies the original underlying cause and the mechanism by which it brings about what troubles you, the unpleasant symptoms from which you seek relief. Whether or not your problem is named and its cause identified, you can and should talk about symptomatic relief with your doctor. Competent physicians aren't offended when their patients get second opinions; feel free to do so if you're in doubt about a diagnosis or recommended treatment.

Decide at the end of each visit if you and your physician will continue to be partners in undertaking your cure. Your orthopedic, neurological, muscular, and medical makeup intersect with the activities of daily life when you have low back pain. The all-inclusive nature of backache makes it essential that you demand and receive the best possible medical care, and that you do your own quality control.

CHAPTER 3

Professional Help

WHEN AND WHOM

T his book is intended to help you develop an idea of what's wrong with your back and decide who should treat your problem. Before contacting someone, however, it's important to consider whether seeing a professional is even necessary.

Is a Professional Necessary?

It may sound odd, but nearly a third of the patients who make an appointment and come to my office want to know nothing more than whether they need to see a doctor. These well-meaning individuals are sincerely trying to take responsibility for themselves, but the luxury of not knowing isn't one that's going to continue to be available in many current health plans. Also, this can waste everybody's time, money, and expertise. Responsible physicians are called on to look carefully at any patient who presents him or herself, and sometimes in the process perform unnecessary tests.

GOOD REASONS FOR SEEKING HELP

Deciding whether you need a doctor need not be difficult. There are four basic rules-of-thumb for seeking help. If any of them applies, or if your pain persists for ten days to two weeks without any reinjury, it's wise to pick up the phone and make an appointment with the practitioner this book should help you choose.

1. Unbearable Pain   The first and most obvious reason for seeing a doctor is that your symptoms are insufferable. They prevent you from concentrating on anything else. It could be extreme pain that incapacitates you, or it could be the tingling in both legs that completely disrupts your day. Pain and unwanted sensations aren't the only reasons to take action in your own behalf. If you need to bend every 10 minutes or so but can't because of pain or stiffness, or pain is unbearable only when you have sex, you need medical attention. I advise you to begin with a physiatrist (a doctor of physical medicine and rehabilitation; see page 70).

2. Progressive Symptoms   In general, symptoms that become increasingly intense are ominous. These include persistent or increasing numbness, weakness, swelling, or abnormal temperature, and persistent skin redness of the legs. A change in bowel, bladder, or sexual function that can't be traced to other causes is ominous. I once saw a patient whose right big toe went numb one week and the next week his left big toe followed suit. He urinated more and more often. At first he tried to laugh it off. What was happening didn't really interfere in his work or personal life. Then all his toes began to lose feeling and he understood he needed to find out why. His diabetes was diagnosed in three days. In six weeks his self-monitored blood sugar became normal, and four months later his numbness had disappeared.

If you are experiencing increasing numbness in your legs and or feet and your control of bowel and/or bladder function is reduced, you should see a neurologist (page 71) or neurosurgeon. If you have a combination of symptoms such as fever, waking up at night in a sweat, numbness or weakness, and in addition you have back pain, you should see an internist (page 70) or rheumatologist (page 73), who can examine you for generalized conditions as well as address your back pain.

3. Chronic Pain   When pain seems unlikely to go away, do something about it. For a while you can ignore an intermittent, mysterious pain, but when the weeks stretch into more than a month, you shouldn't continue to ignore it. Nor should you try to avoid dealing with a pain that you've had before but is worse now than ever before.

A friend of mine used to lift his son's 50-pound barbell every once in a while—despite the pain it always produced for a few days afterward—just to make sure he was still as strong as he'd always been. Then one time he pressed that weight and his back wouldn't quit punishing him for his foolishness. "A week stretched into two weeks, and now into three, and it hasn't gone away," he told me on the phone one night. I had to advise him to come in to my office to see what, if any, damage he'd done.

I'll have more to say about pain, both acute and chronic, in Chapters 4 and 5.

4. Deadline for Relief   There are times people can't wait to ease the pain of a backache. Vacations are planned, or presentations are due at work. Let a doctor examine you when your symptoms aren't insufferable, they have no ominous aspect, and they might go away—if the doctor might provide a good, simple cure. Sometimes two physical therapy sessions, a back brace, or some other uncomplicated, inexpensive measure can speed up recovery or provide relief.

When It's Unnecessary to Seek Help

Just as there are good reasons to seek professional help, there are bad reasons. Sometimes patients come in and ask me to check their backs, not because they have pain or other symptoms, but because they're about to do something they're afraid will produce pain. If you have no history of low back pain or any structural abnormality, an M.D.

can't really tell you with certainty whether your plans are dangerous. A telephone call or a few moments' contemplation may be all that's needed to decide whether superstition may be playing some role. A woman who had suffered a slipped disk while weeding her garden twenty years ago couldn't stifle her urge to call me both before and after every trip to her country home.

A checkup, regardless of how much fear there is that something is wrong, is uncalled for unless there are symptoms. Nor is a visit to the doctor necessary if you know your back pain is really a result of something else that's going on in your life, like increasing generalized fatigue, depression, or physical inflexibility. For fatigue and depression, you may need a few days of vacation and / or a look at circumstances that could affect your physical well-being. And patients who notice increasing lack of body flexibility usually need nothing more than to pay closer attention to their range of motion in a stretch class with an ethical Yoga practitioner or at the local Y or health club.

Medical versus Nonmedical, Western versus Eastern

Let's assume you've considered the reasons for seeking help and decided that indeed you do need to see someone. The question of whom to see can be daunting. Specialists from many different disciplines—medical and nonmedical, Western and Eastern—treat low back pain. This dizzying array becomes even more confusing when taking into consideration that many disciplines have different branches, which may overlap.

You may say to yourself, "I have a bad back. I'll go to an osteopath." But an osteopath can be a general surgeon, a psychiatrist, a pediatrician, or an orthopedist (probably your best choice of the four). Or you may decide you need a massage therapist. However, not only are there different massage schools, there are different methods within a particular school. And it takes a motivated student to ferret out the distinction between the many branches of Yoga and Shiatsu.

To further complicate matters, there's the team approach. If you go to a pain clinic, for example, several experts will cooperate on your treatment, using each other's feedback to work effectively. You will see at least some of the following in your team: a doctor of physical medicine and rehabilitation, a neurologist, an anestheologist, a physical therapist, an occupational therapist, and/or an orthotist (maker of prescribed shoe inserts and braces).

So where do you start? According to a recent study on physician office visits for low back pain, 56 percent of patients first try the doctors in the fields of family medicine, general internal medicine, and osteopathic family medicine. And more than half of the 25 percent of patients who go to orthopedic surgeons have made that decision themselves, without the recommendation of another doctor.

Generalists are often less adept with back pain than specialists. However, in the last few years managed-care firms have found it quite "cost-effective" to employ general practitioners educated in at least the first line of treatment for common low back pain. That's one reason many residency programs in family practice are paying more attention to training doctors to treat this ailment, which strikes at least half of working-age people each year. A family practitioner can also refer you to other experts.

Whether you begin with a generalist or a specialist, when pain doesn't go away and you must choose a treatment direction, I suggest you begin with individuals who have graduated from medical school and passed postdoctoral specialty board exams.

Chronic pain and personal choice have inspired many patients to experiment with the techniques of nonmedical Eastern and Western

---

Did You Know?

The vast majority of cases of low back pain lasts from a few days to a month at most, but reliable research estimates that more than 2.6 million adults are disabled by chronic low back pain at any given time.

specialists. Before signing on with one of these practitioners, check up on the person. Find out what and how much training an individual has had and how long he or she has been in practice. Is the practitioner certified by a learning institution and licensed by the state? Can you get references?

Here are thumbnail sketches of the specialties that deal with back pain.

Medical Specialties

Internal Medicine and Family Practice   Physicians in both these specialties are primary-care doctors. Usually your primary-care doctor knows you best. You go to a member of either one of these specialties for medical care of diseases of your internal organs. Whether your primary-care physician is an internist or a family practitioner, he or she has training in recognizing and treating back problems, especially those of musculoskeletal origin (see Chapter 5), and can prescribe commonsense treatments. These doctors can also diagnose specific serious illnesses, such as kidney disease and signs of cancer that cause back pain. For a large range of serious and minor causes of back pain, these doctors can refer you to other specialists.

Physiatry (Physical Medicine and Rehabilitation)   This relatively young medical specialty came into its own after World War II, when returning injured soldiers needed new and improved techniques to adapt to civilian life. Physicians in this field help patients recover from disability due to injury or illnesses. They are especially expert in the treatment of problems with nerves, joints, muscles, body movement, and posture.

Physiatrists are known for doing thorough physical examinations. They perform or prescribe tests when necessary and are superior diagnosticians. These doctors are taught to work within a team. They are experts at guiding physical, occupational, and speech therapy, and they oversee the use of pain control techniques like TENS (transcutaneous electrical nerve stimulation) and ultrasound (both described in Chapter 11). Physiatrists don't perform surgery and are less likely than members of other specialties to recommend surgery.

Orthopedic Surgery   When a person has back pain and needs a doctor, usually an orthopedic surgeon is chosen. These specialists have studied problems affecting bones, joints, and related structures. They are well known for treating slipped disks, arthritis, and all sorts of back problems. As their name suggests, they are surgically oriented, but a small number of them are academically affiliated and guide physical therapy with expertise. When having surgery, it's always a good idea to learn the details of the procedure, statistics about the outcome, and what recovery will involve.

Neurology and Neurosurgery   These physicians specialize in treating problems whose origins are in the nervous system. They diagnose and treat everything from sciatica to neuropathy (both conditions affecting nerves), and of course, neurosurgeons can perform surgery. A visit to a neurologist includes an examination of nerves, reflexes, motor and sensory functions, and muscles.

Neurosurgeons can be very successful in the treatment of a slipped or herniated disk (a damaged or broken spinal disk), spinal stenosis (narrowing of the inside of the spinal column; Figure 4), and tumors of the spinal canal. Though surgery for carefully selected patients with a slipped disk has a success rate of over 95 percent, there are a great number of unnecessary back surgeries performed in the United States each year.

Osteopathy   Osteopathy is a branch of medicine that grew out of the study of bones and their related structures. Osteopathic physicians are medical doctors known for treating arthritis and related diseases and for working with patients who have backache, especially when it is chronic.

Andrew Taylor Still, M.D., after identifying the musculoskeletal

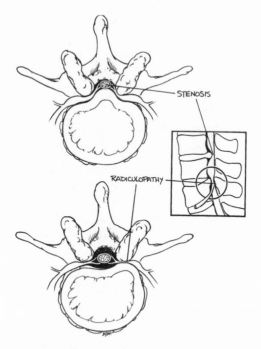

Figure 4. A herniated disk can cause spinal stenosis (narrowing of the spinal canal), shown here. A herniated disk can also press nerve roots as they exit the canal, a condition called radiculopathy.

system as a key element of health, founded the discipline of osteopathy in the late nineteenth century. He based his approach on ideas of preventative medicine and treating the body as a whole. Proper diet, exercise, and fitness are also important to osteopathy. Students of osteopathy are taught body manipulation techniques related to "correct adjustment" of the whole body, including the head.

To become a doctor of osteopathy (D.O.), a student must have an undergraduate degree. Four years of medical school follow, during which studies include all standard medical procedures as well as osteopathic treatments. Upon graduation, D.O.s go on to internships and residencies in osteopathic hospitals or in institutions that employ graduates of conventional medical schools. Osteopaths can specialize in any branch of medicine and become board-certified in that specialty. Optional specialty training, in orthopedics, for example, takes two to six years. Like physicians with M.D. degrees, osteopaths must pass state licensing exams.

Rheumatology   Joints are the main focus of rheumatology, a subspecialty of internal medicine. These physicians treat a wide range of illness involving joints, from gout (painful accumulations of normal proteins near joints) to rheumatoid arthritis (progressive joint damage due to immune system attack). The great advances in immunology have extended the legitimate concerns of rheumatologists to include lupus erythematosus and many other immune or autoimmune processes. When low back pain is caused by arthritis or lupus, a rheumatologist who will address the underlying disease process is helpful.

Anesthesiology   These physicians frequently further specialize in pain management, for which treatment is invasive but not frankly surgical. When other methods or surgery have failed, anaesthesiologists can administer a range of pain-controlling injections. Also, they may work in pain management programs to ease chronic, intractible pain with the use of subcutaneous devices that "mask" painful stimuli.

Podiatry   Foot problems and gait changes are often associated with low back pain. After seeing a family physician or physiatrist, a foot specialist may offer valuable help. Podiatrists have studied the structure and movement of the feet. Some of their services include prescribing orthotics (shoe modification or brace), performing foot surgery, and taking care of problems in the relationship between feet and shoes. They don't have M.D. or D.O. degrees, but they do often affiliate with hospitals. Four years of training are needed to get a degree in podiatry; specialty residencies are available thereafter, frequently in the same hospitals that maintain residencies for medical doctors or osteopathy.

Nonmedical Specialties

ORIENTAL TECHNIQUES

Yoga   The study of Yoga includes meditation, breathing, and other exercises. The Hatha (physical) portion of this ancient Indian philosophical system uses body movements, stretches, and postures to keep practitioners healthy and supple—and is especially helpful for victims of back pain. The stretching and strengthening movements, which should be taught by a qualified instructor before being done alone at home, can both treat low back pain and prevent its recurrence. Pranayama (breath control) is the Yogic path to relaxation and meditation. This breathing technique is widely applied for stress management and is valuable for dealing with musculoskeletal problems in the back and elsewhere, whether or not they are related to stress. Through physical exercise, meditation, and study, the Yoga process aims to release aspirants from attachment to distracting thoughts and material objects and to reveal a higher reality. It is spiritual but features no particular religion.

As a student of B. K. S. Iyengar in India, I saw the healing aspects of Hatha Yoga in action. Practice of postures and exercises taught students the discipline of pain control; the positions and stretches realigned bones, cured muscle spasm, improved body carriage, and eliminated many individuals' back pain once and for all. Unlike many other types of exercise that involve activity that eventually becomes too repetitive and vigorous (and thus can cause injury), Yoga can be practiced for a lifetime.

Acupuncture   The theory on which acupuncture is based came into being almost four thousand years ago in China and remains basically unchanged today. At the beginning of the twentieth century, Sir William Osler, a Canadian physician who worked at Johns Hopkins Medical School, started using acupuncture to relieve low back pain. This system of pain relief became widely known in 1970 when, during a trip to China, journalist James Reston needed an emergency appendectomy. The surgery was performed using acupuncture as anesthesia. Since then, acupuncture has gained steadily in popularity and is now used for a variety of back ailments as well other conditions and even for the control of smoking and other addictions.

According to the basic premise of acupuncture, there are twelve energy channels or meridians and at least four hundred and sixty specific acupuncture points on the human body. These meridians are associated with the lungs, large intestine, stomach, spleen, heart, small intestine, bladder, kidney, gall bladder, and liver. The goal is to deal with physical diseases and conditions by making corrections in the amount of energy in these meridians.

Acupuncturists insert needles into the appropriate points and then manipulate the needles with hands, heat, and other techniques to try to make those corrections. Treatment sessions last up to forty-five minutes, and it generally takes between four and six sessions to assess the result.

Stainless-steel acupuncture needles are not hollow like hypodermic needles, and they can't be used for injections. The needles are flexible, fine (about the thickness of a hair), and so can be inserted with little or no discomfort. Reusable acupuncture needles must be sterilized according to government guidelines, and presterilized disposable needles have become popular with practitioners eager to eliminate the risks of contagion.

Acupuncture is used not only as an anesthetic but for stress management, tennis elbow and other types of tendonitis, "frozen" shoulder, arthritis and joint problems, and many other conditions. While there is no definitive explanation for why acupuncture works, scientists have documented that the manipulation of the needles produces some of the neurophysiological changes associated with morphine and other painkillers. Still, scientific studies remain inconclusive about the success of acupuncture for curing low back pain.

There are many schools of acupuncture in the United States, and training typically takes three to four years. Before admission to most of these institutions, students must learn Western anatomy, physiology, and chemistry. Though some states don't regulate the practice of acupuncture, many require licensing or limit practice only to licensed medical doctors with the proper acupuncture training.

Shiatsu   This traditional Japanese massage therapy done with fingertips is based on ancient Chinese ideas and is an outgrowth of acupuncture. While Shiatsu is aimed at prevention rather than cure, at general well-being rather than at treating specific ailments, it is also used to reduce pain, especially the pain of muscular tension, arthritis, and deep tissue and bone bruises.

Shiatsu diagnosis consists of hands-on examination of the patient's abdomen and other tissues. Treatment includes little massage per se, but concentrates on pressure applied to specific locations, particularly the patient's problem areas. The fully clothed patient lies on the floor or other hard surface to receive this therapy, which is not meant to be painful. Active and passive exercises and stretching may be part of the treatment.

Acupressure   This massage technique relies on pressure applied with the therapist's fingertips, knuckles, or a special tool called a "Tei Shin." Depending on the practitioner, there are thirty to forty acupressure points, some corresponding to those of Shiatsu. The goal of this therapy is to increase circulation and release physical and emotional tension.

Learning from an accupressure therapist, patients can find it relatively easy to use this technique themselves for relief of muscle spasm and other musculoskeletal difficulties. Pressure, applied by therapist or patient, can relax tight muscles and reduce pain.

WESTERN TECHNIQUES

Chiropractic   Second in size only to the medical health-care system, chiropractic is the most popular avenue for people seeking relief from low back pain. Surveys show that more than 70 percent of people suffering from chronic back pain visit chiropractors nearly twice as often as physicians in a given year.

Chiropractors believe that the relationship between structure and function in the human body is a significant health factor and that links between the spinal column and the nervous system contribute to disease processes.

The best-known treatment method chiropractors use is structural adjustment. This hands-on manipulation is aimed at correcting subluxated (out-of-place) spinal or pelvic segments and relieving associated nerve, muscle, and vascular disturbances. Practitioners also use taping, strapping, and braces to assist healing and prevent reinjury. They can order and read X rays and have admitting and treatment privileges in many hospitals. The American Medical Association sanctions referrals to doctors of chiropractic by M.D.s, and many health insurance policies cover chiropractic.

To become a chiropractor, a student must complete a minimum of two years of college and four academic years of professional training. In order to practice in all states, graduates must pass a licensing board examination and the Basic Science Board Examination required for M.D.s and doctors of osteopathy.

A 1994 Harris poll found that the public feels chiropractors are the most effective specialists for treating low back problems. While I agree that chiropractors and other nonmedical experts can and do effectively treat back pain, I suspect that lower cost, office informality, and the ease of getting appointments had as much to do with these survey results as the actual effectiveness of chiropractic—to say nothing of the fact that a great deal of backache disappears by itself.

Physical Therapy   Physiatrists and other physicians, most frequently those in nonsurgical specialties, prescribe physical therapy for patients who are recovering from an injury or have back pain. Physical therapy is widely used to prevent or reduce joint stiffness, to restore muscle strength, and to reduce pain, inflammation, and spasm. It is often extremely successful for patients who have back pain of musculoskeletal as well as neurological origins.

Physical therapists have been trained in the use of a wide range of hands-on techniques, among them massage, manipulation, application of heat and cold, postural instruction, relaxation, and exercise. They also know how to apply ultrasound, electrical muscle stimulation, and TENS. These techniques are described in greater detail in Chapter 11.

During a physical therapy session, a patient might receive passive stretching (be moved by the therapist), learn how to contract and relax certain muscle groups to relieve spasm and increase strength, and how to perform certain movements so that an injury is not aggravated. The number of sessions a patient needs depends on the original condition and progress.

Physical therapists help patients assess and correct problems in their environments or activities of daily living, such as adjusting a desk that is too high or altering bad posture. Some stress management also falls into their domain. Their approach is individualized, so they can treat seriously disabled patients who need to be seen at home as well as patients with mild, passing problems.

In many states people can go directly to a physical therapist without seeing a physician first.

Manual Medicine   This method of manipulation, which is based on anatomy and kinesiology (the mechanics of movement), started as a separate specialty in Europe in the 1980s and has since developed a following here in the United States. It involves knowing how joints can and do move during normal daily activity. By applying pressure and using limbs and joints themselves as levers and fulcrums to produce greater force, therapists reposition, loosen, or mobilize joints and muscles. Physical therapists and osteopaths use fingertips to achieve myofascial release (manual separation of muscle tissue to loosen connective tissue), making muscles more responsive, mobile, and less painful. In the application of strain/counterstrain techniques, patients cooperate to use their own muscle power and bone length for necessary repositioning, for example, in adjusting the sacroiliac joint. Manual medicine overlaps with other disciplines, including chiropractic, osteopathy, physical therapy, and shiatsu and acupressure, but it isn't the same as any one of them.

Biofeedback   This technique is said to assist patients in regulating their own stress levels, pain, and other (usually involuntary) physical processes and responses. Electrodes that measure some pain-related feature such as muscle tension are attached at one end to the patient and at the other end to a machine that monitors the response and emits a sound or visual signal. The signal is the feedback, a reading of the particular reaction, such as muscle tension. The biofeedback therapist's goal is to teach the patient, through concentration and methods related to meditation, to control the machine's signal, and by extension to control his or her own body process.

Biofeedback training is usually conducted by a health-care professional. It is used for treatment of chronic pain, muscle spasm, vascular problems such as Reynaud's syndrome, and general relaxation training. As of this writing, there were no major studies showing that biofeedback can relieve or cure low back pain. The National Institutes of Health (NIH), in conjunction with licensed members of the Association for Applied Psychophysiology and Biofeedback, are currently exploring the possibility with one thousand subjects.

Hypnosis   In spite of its murky reputation as a parlor game or an evil form of mind control, hypnosis has been proven useful for pain alleviation and for behavior modification, including stress management. Major surgery, even leg amputation, has been performed under hypnosis, but this technique is considered most effective when used to relieve pain from muscle tension and psychological causes.

Subjects are put into a "trance" state, an attentive, relaxed and receptive form of consciousness. Though scientists don't know exactly how hypnosis works on a physiological level, there is no doubt that suggestions made by the hypnotist to the subject have a great deal to do with the success of the outcome.

Twenty years ago, physicians in the pain clinic at Walter Reed Army Medical Center used hypnosis on more than half their patients, endorsing it as beneficial, relatively cheap, and nonaddictive. Today, the Office of Alternative Medicine at the NIH, in conjunction with Virginia Polytechnic Institute and State University, is conducting a small study to see how analgesia (pain relief) through hypnotic suggestion affects the electrophysiology of specific regions of the brain in nondepressed patients with low back pain.

Swedish Massage   This is the type of massage best known to the public and popular in health clubs and spas. And no wonder. Having a Swedish massage is a relaxing, pleasurable experience. Somewhat vigorous, hands-on manipulation has the basic effect of improving circulation briefly. It can relieve back pain of musculoskeletal origin, reduce stiffness and swelling, lower stress level, and provide the subject with a sense of well-being. Along with other types of massage, it is a staple for athletes.

The Swedish massage therapist usually works on the subject over most of the body, using oil or lotion to make the hands glide more easily on the skin. The technique, which grew out of the work of Per Hendrik Ling (1776–1839), consists of several different manipulations, including stroking, kneading, tapping, rubbing, and creating vibrations. A full-body massage generally lasts thirty to sixty minutes. In my experience with patients, these massages are more pleasant than therapeutic. Though they may not completely cure a backache, they rarely do the subject any harm.

Go to a Swedish massage therapist who has a license. There are many handbooks for people interested in learning Swedish massage, and they can be of use if you decide to practice it yourself with a mate or friend.

Alexander Technique   Matthias Alexander (1869–1955) was an actor with cervical pain. He developed a method to help students observe and change muscular habits and posture that seemed to interfere with optimum function. Classes in the Alexander technique are popular among actors and dancers, and are considered useful for people with back problems. Students learn a series of simple but subtle movements designed to increase awareness of tension and behavior patterns and to change those that are detrimental. The goal of the Alexander technique is to help students unlearn responses and actions that lead to tension and pain. This system is meant to be used to help practitioners achieve physical and mental well-being.

Feldenkrais Method   The Feldenkrais method is based on the idea that, in the natural course of events, individuals learn just enough to function but not to function at an optimum level. Its creator, Moshe Feldenkrais (1904–1984), believed in improving basic functional skills like walking. The method uses manipulation and exercise to achieve better posture, flexibility, and coordination and to produce muscle relaxation.

Students of the Feldenkrais method learn functional integration through hands-on work with an instructor. Lying on a table, fully and comfortably clothed, the instructor guides the student through a series of movements designed to break bad habits and retrain the nervous system. Group lessons, called Awareness through Movement, consist of slow physical exercises.

Instructors must graduate from a Feldenkrais Guild accredited program, a process that usually takes four years.

Pilates   Joseph Pilates, a Greek gymnast, believed people need balancing, control, alignment, and centering to be healthy and pain-free. With this in mind, shortly after World War II he designed equipment with springs to facilitate exercise and postural adjustment. Pushing against spring resistance, students work to increase muscle flexibility, tone, and length. Pilates is popular with athletes, dancers, and many people with back problems. All students work first in private sessions with instructors, who aid them in using the equipment and address individual problems; then students attend semiprivate sessions. Training certification as an instructor in Pilates is done under the auspices of the Physical Mind Institute in Santa Fe, New Mexico, and takes about a year.

Rolfing   Rolfing is an emotional as well as a physical therapy system developed by Ida P. Rolf, Ph.D. (1896–1979), who was influenced by the Alexander technique, osteopathy, Yoga, and Gestalt therapy (a form of psychotherapy using role playing). The goal of Rolf's therapy is to balance the patient's body in gravity through manipulation, and to restore elasticity to hardened, stiffened, or thickened connective tissue.

The Rolfing system addresses chronic muscular tension and shortened muscle linings resulting from poor posture, disease, physical trauma, repetitive injury syndrome, surgery, and emotional distress, as well as environmental factors such as ill-fitting shoes and beds. Rolfers approach the body in blocks, striving for proper alignment. They use fingers, open hands, fists, and elbows to manipulate the subject's major muscle groups and surrounding connective tissue.

Patients report that the treatments can be quite painful, but benefits are said to include pain relief, greater freedom of joint movement, and increased energy, as well as release from emotional trauma, anger, and resentment.

Rolfers are required to have a B.A. or B.S. degree from an accredited college and specialized training that takes about a year to complete.

In the remaining chapters, let's find out what's wrong, and which of these many resources may be right for you.

CHAPTER 4

Pain

ITS FORMS AND NAMES

I n Chapter 3 I touched briefly on pain as a reason for seeking professional help. In this chapter, I hope to familiarize you with some of the fundamental concepts, vocabulary, and causes of back pain. Knowing how to describe and categorize what you're feeling, and having at least a notion about reasons for your problem, are the basis for intelligent action. The idea here isn't to come up with a definitive diagnosis, but to have enough information to form an opinion about whether you need help from a professional, and if you do, from whom.

What Is Pain?

Trying to describe and define pain—and its counterpart, pleasure—has kept philosophers and physicians busy for centuries and has reduced even such brilliant men as Aristotle to babble. Luckily we do have some working definitions.

In 1979 the taxonomy committee of the International Association of the Study of Pain came up with this definition of pain: "an unpleasant sensory and emotional experience associated with actual or potential tissue damage, or described in terms of such damage." And then they made this crucial addition: "Pain is always subjective. Each individual learns the application of the word through experiences related to injury early in life. It is unquestionably a sensation in part of the body, but it is also always unpleasant and therefore also an emotional experience."

We can't feel another person's pain; we can only try to imagine from our own experience what it might be like. Trying to empathize, to put ourselves in the other person's shoes, might lead us to wonder if it's possible for two people to feel the same thing and only one of them to call it painful. At first glance, considering the vast differences in our personalities, bodies, and pain thresholds, the answer seems to be yes. On second thought, if two people are really both experiencing the same thing, they would have the same experience.

Any discussion of pain has to include awareness of the trickiness of the concept.

Symptoms and Signs

Symptoms are what usually bring people in to see health-care workers, and the most common symptom when it comes to back problems is pain. The category of symptoms occupies a broad spectrum, but signs belong in another category that is also crucial to diagnosing what's wrong and deciding on a treatment program.

Pain, numbness, tingling, and anything else you feel subjectively is a symptom. When it comes to symptoms, you're the world's greatest expert, and the examining physician or other clinician wants to hear all about them from you. Objective tests don't measure the ache, the lightning shocks, the sensation of pins and needles. Only you know how intensely or when you feel one of those symptoms, or any other.

It's true that while symptoms are subjective, some also can have objective counterparts. When you cut your finger and see blood flowing out, for example, you know exactly where you feel the pain. Though where you have injured yourself can be seen by everyone, and how serious the injury is can be estimated by its size and amount of bleeding, your subjective judgment is still final. You are the only one who really knows how much that cut hurts, the only one who can express your personal experience in words.

Signs are the opposite of symptoms in that they're objective. Professionals are trained to read these signs. The knocking that physicians do with their reflex hammers, the peeping into your eyes with ophthalmoscopes, the listening for your heartbeat with stethoscopes— all these actions, performed by the keen observer, detect signs such as the absence of a reflex, retinal detachment, weakness, or a creaking, out of kilter joint. Signs are also the results of blood tests, spinal taps, and imaging studies like X rays and MRIs.

The difference between signs and symptoms can be summed up this way: a blood-pressure reading is a sign, but feeling your heart go thump, thump, thump is a symptom.

Of course, some things are a combination of signs and symptoms. For instance, a reflex is an objective phenomenon elicited when a clinician taps a tendon at, for example, your knee. The muscle stretches, initiating a sensory impulse that travels up your spinal cord. This in turn stimulates motor nerves to carry the impulse back down to the muscle above your knee, causing it to contract. The vigor of the response—how strong it is—is a sign. You feel the tap because at the same time sensory nerves also travel to the brain, connecting with higher centers. If you feel it as a heavy blow or a hot wire, that's a symptom.

But what if your nerve has been severed? When the doctor wields his or her hammer, you feel nothing. It might seem that the reason for this lack of response is subjective—your leg remains inert because you can't feel anything. That, however, would be an illusion. If the nerves are intact, the reflex will be too. It will function or not regardless of feeling, and your response to the tap of the hammer will be observable whether you're awake or asleep. When the nerve is cut, the reflex disappears, along with the physiological basis of feeling. The absence of feeling is a symptom. Your body, by reacting or not reacting to a reflex test, gives the clinician a sign.

So, it's important to understand that the objective signs, your subjective symptoms, and your history must all go "into the hopper," before the physician can arrive at a firm opinion about what might be troubling you.

Intensity

How do you know when discomfort or annoyance has turned to pain that needs to be dealt with? The answer is: if what you're feeling interrupts the concentration you need in order to do something, or if it interferes with your enjoyment. When you're aware that a task as simple as making tea has become difficult to perform because of that dull but persistent ache in the small of your back, or you can't really sit still in your favorite chair and comfortably enjoy watching the nightly news, then it's time to take action.

One of the main elements of any painful sensation is that it can vary in intensity. Unlike an object, which you can either see and touch or not, pain has more than two extremes: it can go from slight to moderate, severe, extreme, and finally to unbearable. Since the beginning of time, patients have tried to describe their pain to healers, who have had to use empathy and guesswork to understand. This fundamental difficulty has not been completely resolved. Nevertheless, scientists have taken advantage of the variability of pain by devising a way to analyze it quantitatively even though feeling it is subjective.

The Visual Analog Scale (Figure 5) is a tried-and-true, standard instrument used to quantify pain. It has been tested in a number of contexts and found to be reliable and reproducible. When using this scale, doctors ask patients to "grade" their pain from 1 to 10 on a ruler-like scale, and then measure the pain in millimeters. It can be useful to think of what you feel in the following way:

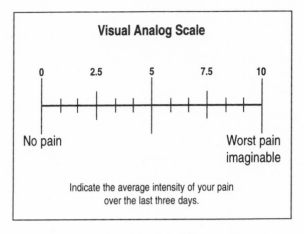

Figure 5. The Visual Analog Scale objectively quantifies pain.

0—no pain at all

2—the sort of thing we may all experience when carrying a heavy bundle a long distance

7—an intense pain that might take the enjoyment out of many daily activities

8 or 9—pain that brings us close to screaming

Studying pain on a numerical scale like this one can give both patients and clinicians a clearer definition of a patient's symptoms. It also provides objective feedback about whether pain relief methods are effective. If your pain usually varies between 5 and 7, and after a few days of taking a new medicine the pain hovers between 2 and 4 and doesn't rise higher, it's likely that the medicine is doing some good, that is, 50 percent of the job. The pain scale can also be used to gauge the effectiveness of physical therapy, acupuncture, or any other technique. And it can measure if and how much your untreated pain changes over time.

Another scale, the Functional Interference Estimate (FIE), developed by Timothy Toomey at the University of North Carolina, provides a simple, straightforward way for you to find out how disabling your pain is by measuring how much it cuts into daily activities.

A third tool for studying pain, the McGill-Melzack Pain Scale (Figure 6), involves using a paper outline of the front and back of a hypothetical person. With a pen or pencil, you can indicate exactly where it hurts and describe the pain by circling any one or a combination of sixty descriptive words. In the future a computerized version of this kind of scale might assist patients by analyzing that information along with other data and then listing possible diagnoses.

Types of Pain

People can and frequently do feel more than one variety of pain at the same time. It's important to be able to characterize pain with the most accurate words possible when you communicate symptoms to health-care workers. But just as crucial as correctly describing symptoms is knowing that certain kinds of pain are often associated with specific difficulties. A discussion of possible diagnoses may seem premature at this point in our study of symptoms, but jumping ahead to a brief discussion of causes of pain may give you an advantage. It makes sense to have information about what types of problems and conditions usually go with the various types of pain so that you can follow along as your physician investigates your case and be of as much help as possible in arriving at a diagnosis.

ACHE

Any part of your body can ache. Generally, however, an ache is a vague, unfocused pain that occurs in a muscular or muscular-bony portion of the body. Aches usually register in the range of 2 to 5 on the pain scale, 5 being an average toothache, which is quite unpleasant but bearable. While this type of pain can vary in intensity, if it

McGill - Melzack Pain Questionnaire

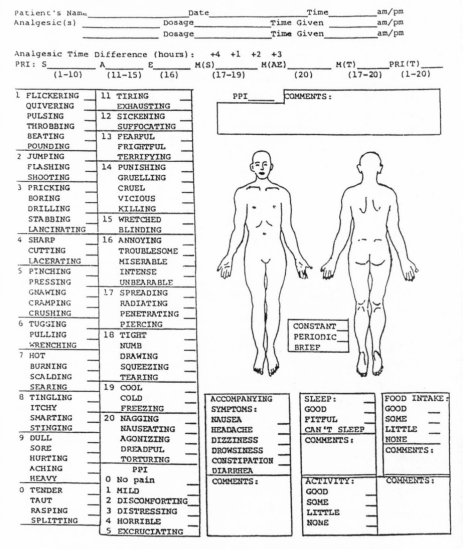

Figure 6. The McGill-Melzack Pain Scale helps locate and characterize pain.

becomes severe, a word other than "ache" defines it more accurately. I've always thought what people call a "splitting headache" would be more aptly described as "a terrible pain in the head." An ache should not alarm you. Of all the types of pain there are, this is the one that is most likely to go away by itself.

Joints (where muscle, tendons, ligaments, and bones connect) sometimes ache, but as I said before, most aches are muscular in nature and origin. Often an ache in a muscle is caused by nothing more than:

1. a sprain (tearing a few fibers of a ligament),
2. a strain (inflammation in a muscle or tendon caused by using it beyond normal range or capacity), or
3. overexertion (which, if unusually high, can cause excessive flow of blood into the muscles, producing an ache by painfully distending the tiny capillaries inside).

BURNING

A painful burn can of course be caused by fire, acid, or other chemicals or friction. But a person can experience a burning sensation over large or small portions of the body when no such injury has occurred. Unless there is clear and visible injury to the skin, a burning sensation is generally neurological. When associated with problems of the back, a burning feeling frequently goes from being a very mild, just barely suspected sensation to the point of being utterly intolerable. It can be continuous for long periods of time.

Many types of neurological problems cause burning sensations, which are a common form of back pain. A pinched nerve root high in the cervical spine can result in headache and a burning sensation on the skin of the neck, arms, and hands. In the lumbar spine, a pinched nerve root can produce the same symptoms, but lower down: on the trunk, lower back, buttocks, genital area, legs, and feet. A burning sensation can also be caused by pinched nerves elsewhere in

the body, and you may feel it days or weeks after the injury has occurred. A trauma can make a nerve vulnerable to innocuous stimuli,
like almost weightless clothing brushing against skin.

Injury to the outer coverings of nerves disrupts the way impulses
travel, producing something like telephone-wire interference and
causing bizarre feelings, some of which people describe as "burning."
A knife wound or an injury that crushes a nerve can cause this, as can
piriformis syndrome and carpal tunnel syndrome (which results when
the median nerve is compressed at the wrist, causing pain in the
thumb, fingers, and hand).

These aren't the only causes of a burning sensation. A neuropathy, in which one or more nerves are functioning abnormally because of a systemic or regional body condition, can also result in this
unpleasant type of pain. Neuropathies can be caused by diabetes,
chemotherapy, alcoholism, heredity, and a host of other factors, even
from overdoses of certain vitamins.

ELECTRIC SHOCK

When your finger makes contact with a light socket, many different
nerve fibers are stimulated simultaneously. Some of these fibers communicate temperature, others the motion of joints and muscles. The
nervous system registers this unpleasant overload of various sensations as electric shock. You feel this on the skin of your fingertip and
all the way up your arm.

A similar phenomenon occurs at the moment a nerve, with all its
various fibers, is suddenly squeezed or compressed. Many nerves of
various types discharge all at once. When you have a pinched nerve
in your lower back, you usually feel radiating pain traveling down
along the path of the sciatic nerve, sometimes all the way to the skin
of the foot.

While a person can experience almost constant electric shock–like
pains over a period of hours, each little episode is structured in that
it has a beginning, a middle, and an end. Another typical aspect of this

pain is that the lightninglike electric shocks usually travel from the point of occurrence away from the spinal cord.

Electric shocks travel along the path of a nerve and usually involve that nerve or its origins. The site of the injury, however, doesn't have to be in that nerve or the nerves that connect to it. In some instances, a brain tumor, multiple sclerosis, syphilis, or all forms of meningitis can be the cause of the sensation of electric shocks. They can also come from diabetic or other neuropathies.

Frequently electric shock–like pains come and go according to various factors such as position, pressure, or lifting heavy objects. Reaching into the overhead compartment of an airplane, for instance, might cause shocks down the legs. Pressure from outside, like hitting your funny bone or sitting too long can make you vulnerable to this type of pain, as can pressure from inside, like coughing or laughing. A structural pathology like a radiculopathy is the most common cause of this unpleasant sensation.

GNAWING

This pain is difficult to distinguish from an ache. Like an ache, a gnawing pain can originate in a muscle. Unlike an ache that occupies the entire volume of an area, however, a gnawing pain may occupy only the edges. Gnawing pains are frequently but not necessarily mild.

A characteristic of gnawing pains is that they seem to be progressive even when they are not. One cause of this kind of sensation is cancer, where there is literally an eating away or a progressive disruption and displacement of tissue. Myopathy—a primary, often hereditary and fairly unusual disease affecting muscle tissue—can also cause a gnawing sensation.

Perhaps one of the most unpleasant aspects of gnawing pain is emotional. The pain seems as if it's going to progress, but it often doesn't. It's not as if a mouse were actually gnawing at a slice of cheese, first nibbling at the right corner, then at the middle or somewhere else. People who experience gnawing pain may feel it always in the same spot, but it seems as if it's going to go further. That may cause fear and dread, usually unwarranted emotions.

STABBING

This type of pain can be just as sudden, intense, and structured as the neurological sensation of electric shock, though usually the pain is visceral or muscular rather than directly involving a nerve. Stabbing pains are caused by a kidney stone, for example, or a gall-bladder attack. You know instinctively when a stabbing pain reaches its peak and when it starts to fade. Though it may repeat, it rarely occurs again and again in rapid succession. Very infrequently do people complain of what happened to St. Sebastian, who may have survived many arrow wounds and multiple stabbing pains in various parts of the body. Usually patients come to me with stabbing pains that may be repetitive but not incessant; sometimes these pains do have a neurological component that causes the sensation of burning in addition to stabbing. That can happen with piriformis syndrome, a type of sciatica in which there is a stab in the buttock and the back of the thigh and burning of the outside of the calf.

TWISTING

This is another pain that has its origins in the nerves. You feel as if someone is grasping your skin, turning it and stretching it at the same time, or that someone is wringing a whole limb, all the muscles and joints, and putting some rotational pressure on the bone too. Twisting can be a type of phantom pain. Studies have found that if a nerve is stimulated and then severed, the place that nerve came from in the spinal cord or brain stem can continue its activity for quite a length of time, sometimes for years. Patients who have had a leg amputated, either above or below the knee, can therefore "feel" a twisting or crushing pain in the missing big toe (see Chapter 7).

MECHANICAL TENSION: CRUSHING, PINCHING, SQUEEZING, OR PULLING

These four sensations are really of pressure rather than pain per se. A feeling of crushing can of course be brought on simply by too much weight on a part of the body. An example would be if you stepped barefoot on a marble and all your body weight were concentrated on that one small area of skin. In this case, the crushing pain is felt in the bones of the ball of the foot. Muscle spasm, especially in the hips or lower back, can produce any one of these four sensations.

Another cause of pain from mechanical tension is when a body structure meant to protect other structures is injured by their movement. When swollen, after even mild trauma, a bursa that should separate a muscle and bone, or a tendon, muscle, and bone, can cause a crushing pain. In a situation like this, the irritated bursa can swell, and the more it swells, the more it gets in the way of the muscle and the more injury it sustains. What you have then is a vicious cycle.

Generally, nature has taken adequate steps to make sure that two inner structures moving by one another can slide smoothly, without hampering each other's movement in any way. Like everything else, this breaks down from time to time. Adhesions, for instance, are connections between usually separate structures that may form in the process of healing after an operation or injury. Between two muscles or two moving body parts like the folds of the shoulder joints or layers of tissue in the abdomen, adhesions can cause pinching, squeezing, pulling, or crushing pains.

The sensations of pinching, crushing, or squeezing can also occur when a tendon or part of a joint capsule gets trapped at a place where there's a small joint and a big range of motion, like the shoulder. Consider what happens when you raise your arm over your head: The tissue around the joint capsule, folded down when not in use, stretches out like a fan. It can get pinched between two bones—in the case of the shoulder, between the humerus and the scapula. This produces a severe compression and crushing pain.

THROBBING

In 99 out of 100 cases this unpleasant sensation has a definite repetitive rhythm like a heartbeat. In the back the problem isn't cardiac (relating to the heart), but in all likelihood it is inflammatory or vascular (relating to circulation). If you've got a big bruise, for instance, the reason for the throbbing is fairly simple: Expanded and distended blood vessels literally bump into swollen, inflamed tissue. Nerve-stimulating chemicals resulting from inflammation amplify the throbbing sensation.

An aneurism (an opening in a vein or artery, like a weak place in a garden hose which produces a bulging and thinning of the tube) is an example of a vascular problem that could cause throbbing. Another cause of throbbing is when an artery takes an anatomical "shortcut" to a vein. This starts when a tiny channel between an artery and vein widens because of pressure. Some or even almost all the blood from the artery passes through this shortcut. Because the blood is not making the usually lengthier journey through tiny capillaries, the pulse is not damped down and the vein throbs. More blood passing through the shortcut makes the vein throb more.

Throbbing is usually in the location of the problem or injury. Of course, high blood pressure can cause throbbing, but generally only in the head or chest.

EMOTION-PRODUCING PAIN

Any of the types of pains I've described can have emotional aspects. Pain can be punishing, frightening, depressing, and isolating. It can make you feel guilty, remorseful, powerless, or angry. And, of course, by its very nature, pain has its own emotional component. When emotions run high, it is usually of great value to recognize that they will vanish when the pain does. Unwanted emotions associated with pain can but don't always help motivate patients to seek diagnosis and cure. Don't neglect to tell your physician if your pain is accompanied by strong emotion. It's an important aspect of your symptoms.

Pain can be wearing. It can depress and discourage you and negatively affect your view of the world. It can also provide knowledge
and the motivation to take action aimed at change. As Sophocles said
2,400 years ago, "For all calamities save death itself, man has found
ways to help."

S C I A T I C A

Sciatica hurts, but it isn't an illness. This pain, like all others, is a
symptom. If sciatica continues, chances are the cause will too, and it
might be necessary to look for it. It has been shown that most sciatica comes from a pinched nerve somewhere in the lower lumbar
spine, but it can also originate in the piriformis muscle or the sacroiliac joint, which we'll discuss in detail later in Chapter 9.

You feel the pain of sciatica along the anatomical path of the sciatic nerve and its branches, from the lumbar spine through the buttock, down the back of the leg and calf to the sole of the foot or big
toe (Figure 7). It can be constant or intermittent. The pain is sometimes a straightforward, garden-variety ache, or it can be unpleasant
sensations of electric shock, heat, tingling, or stabbing pain. It can take
many forms, sometimes changing in character during a single day.

With any pain, and particularly with sciatica, it's useful to look for
a pattern. What is its character, how does it change? What makes it
start? Can you make it stop, even briefly? Does it have anything to do
with position or time of day? With intermittent sciatica, ask yourself
what adaptations you can make to relieve the pain.

If sciatica causes disability or is accompanied by weakness, numbness, unusual swelling, or alteration of bowel, bladder, or sexual functions, it needs medical attention. Obviously, extraordinary pain also
calls for immediate treatment by a professional.

Both constant and intermittent sciatic pain may be due to a herniated disk, arthritis severe enough to constrict the space through
which the roots of this nerve must pass, a tumor, or other com-

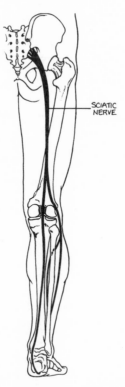

SCIATIC
NERVE

Figure 7. Pain and other symptoms of sciatica can appear anywhere along the path of the sciatic nerve.

plaints. Pain that changes in type and location may be the symptom of a structural problem, like spinal stenosis or sacroiliac joint derangement. When intermittent pain comes from an activity like jogging or sitting too long, it can be difficult to diagnose. A combination of small functional and structural abnormalities often doesn't show up on tests, so diagnosis is more dependent on a full physical examination. Diabetes, osteoporosis, and other metabolic problems also can cause sciatica.

Patients are often confused about sciatica. They think it's a diagnosis. That's not correct. Sciatica, as said before, is a symptom. It may

---

DID YOU KNOW?

Sciatica is one of three main clinical categories for low back pain, according to the Agency for Health Care Policy and Research, *Clinical Practice Guideline*, number 14. The other two are potentially serious spinal conditions and nonspecific back symptoms.

---

be accompanied by other signs or symptoms that lead to a diagnosis and plan for treatment.

Diagnostic Clues

Paying close attention to pain and observing it in all the aspects you can think of will increase your chances for quickly arriving at a diagnosis and cure. Here are some factors you should note carefully and pass along to your doctor, if you need to see one. Please remember that the possible causes linked with symptoms in the examples below are not all-inclusive, but are meant to lead you in the right direction by ruling out some factors and focusing the investigation. In general, a pattern of pain and symptoms is extremely useful to a doctor trying to arrive at a diagnosis.

TIME OF DAY

Rheumatoid arthritis (an immune system disorder) pain is usually felt in the morning, while osteoarthritis (degenerative joint disease) causes more pain after activity and as the day progresses.

EXERCISE

Exercise can cause pain in several ways. Movement, pressure, and weight bearing create pain in a broken bone. Sometimes, however, when pain is associated with movement, there is nothing structurally wrong. In other words, an MRI wouldn't show a problem, but the pain could come from internal parts not moving in smooth coordination with one another. As I said earlier, a bone rubbing against a bursa can cause trouble, for example, as can legs differing in length by as little as three-eighths of an inch.

Painful muscle fatigue from exercise often arises from vascular problems that prevent enough oxygen and glucose from reaching the muscles and retard removal of the acidic waste products produced in the muscle as it works. This symptom is called intermittent claudication. Still another functional cause of pain during exercise is improper position or movement, which results in excessive stress on joints, muscles, or other tissues. An example of this is a blister that formed on the palm of your hand while you mowed the lawn. There's nothing wrong with the lawn mower and nothing wrong with your hand. It was the improper interaction that caused the blister. Sometimes these improper interactions are more than skin deep; for example, new mothers sometimes hurt their backs by picking up the baby without lowering the side of the crib.

POSITION

A straight torso either standing up or lying down aggravates the pain caused by spinal stenosis; a bent or curved spine relieves that pain but intensifies pain in patients with a radiculopathy or piriformis syndrome. Lying "upside down," with head and shoulders lower than the rest of the body, relieves back pain in pelvic conjestion syndrome (a circulatory problem, primarily in women, that results in swelling). Some car seats put the driver in a position that almost inevitably causes sciatic pain when feet are used on brake and gas pedals.

COUGHING OR SNEEZING

Increased pressure inside the spinal column may cause pain when there is a herniated disk, or when the patient suffers from spinal stenosis or a tumor.

PAIN WITH SPECIFIC ACTIVITIES

If your lower back hurts when you swing your legs into or out of a car, the problem is likely in the sacroiliac joint. A herniated disk, "facet syndrome,"[1] mildly displaced ribs, or simple muscle pain can make it more difficult to turn in one direction than the other.

Pain that gets worse when you walk can be caused by intermittent claudication. Pain when walking can also be caused by spinal stenosis, since when we walk our backs are quite erect. Victims of these conditions can experience impotence, leg weakness, and sensory changes.

If standing still eliminates pain in a matter of seconds, the cause is vascular. If lying flat brings on pain, your problem is likely spinal stenosis, though pain while lying down frequently occurs when a patient has prostate or other cancer. If sitting makes you miserable, the cause might be in sacroiliac joint disease, ischial bursitis, radiculopathy, or piriformis syndrome.

Pain is nature's way of letting you know something is wrong; it often helps you find out what the problem is. However, sometimes pain itself is the only serious problem, and once you deal with the pain, the underlying cause needs no further attention. Still, knowing the cause is critical in deciding how to proceed. Analyzing your pain will lead you to its source. In Chapter 5 I discuss how to conduct your own investigation.

---

[1]Many believe one lumbar facet can hook behind another. I have never seen X-ray, CT scan, or MRI confirmation of this.

Musculoskeletal Pain

WHERE IT HURTS AND WHY

Location, location, location explains 85 percent of all back pain. When I say "location," I refer to muscles as well as specific regions of the spine. Incredibly, most medical schools spend more than a month studying the cells and biochemistry of the liver and less than an hour on all the different muscles of the back. Without going through four years of medical school, reading the following pages should help you identify and (when necessary) treat

---

DID YOU KNOW?

According to a recent study, doctors diagnose "nonspecific backache" for 56 percent of patients who come to them with low back pain. This diagnosis really means musculoskeletal problems, including strains, sprains, lumbago (sacroiliac joint pain is one definition of this archaic term), and backache caused by stress and other emotional problems.

---

muscle problems or mechanical malfunctions in your lower back.

Thankfully, pain that is musculoskeletal in origin may very well go away by itself or respond to noninvasive treatment. Of course, your age, your condition, and the severity of the injury will all contribute to the length of time you hurt. No matter how long that is, drugstore medications, massage, and swimming or gentle exercise like Yoga will relieve stiffness resulting from overexercise and mild spasm.

If the pain isn't musculoskeletal but is due to abnormalities in your back, time is a clue. Musculoskeletal pain usually goes away in a relatively short time. If your pain persists for more than two weeks, or continues to interfere with your daily activities for that long, you should consult a physician.

Where the Pain Is

I'm going to concentrate now on low back pain, but bear in mind that your neck, shoulders, ribs, spine behind the ribs—all these can hurt because of your body's adaptation to low back pain. When the lower and upper back begin to hurt at the same time, it's usually for the same reason. Frequently pain comes from musculoskeletal difficulties, including sprain, strain, spasm, and/or mechanical problems.

The lumbar spine begins where the ribs leave off and continues down to the sacrum and coccyx. As explained in Chapter 1, this part of the backbone is less fixed and more flexible than the thoracic spine because it lacks the rigid support of the ribs. This design provides for movement and is a counterpart to the more or less immovable, weight-bearing pelvis. Still, the lumbar spine is less flexible than the neck, for it has a major weight-bearing function (Figure 8).

Because of our ability to move our lower and upper extremities separately, our lumbar spines bear much of the burden of our support. The well-being of this part of the backbone depends on strength, posture, coordination, and balance. While muscles provide support, the position and carriage of the body as a whole are essen-

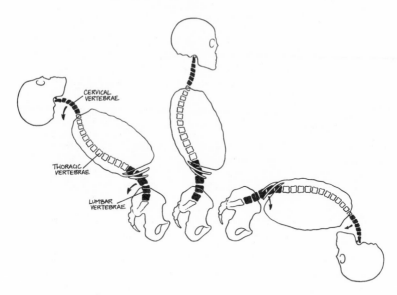

Figure 8.   The lumbar spine has less mobility and more stability; the cervical spine is more mobile but less stable.

tial for balancing weight, for resisting the pull of gravity, and for withstanding forces that movement generates on spinal structures.

Before delving deeper into the anatomy of the spine, recall again that the lower back is part of a major support and communications structure that connects your head to your "tail." The seven cervical vertebrae of the neck, the 12 thoracic vertebrae to which the ribs are connected, and even the head itself, can cause low back pain. Often pain in these areas that begins simultaneously with low back pain, or shows up the day after, reflects a problem with posture. Adapting to the pain may have made it awkward to reach for the telephone receiver, roll down a car window, or walk normally, but the pain in the thoracic or cervical regions vanishes when low back pain has been treated correctly. The position of the neck above the back makes neck pain the subject of another book. However, when the pain in the lower back disappears along with the pain in the neck, you know they had the same cause.

Look for a Pattern

You wake up one morning and your lower back hurts. It's like a dull ache, really, but more severe, and it gets worse when you press on the small of your back, where the source of pain seems to be. You're afraid you're not going to be able to move, but within a few minutes you're creakily sitting up and easing yourself out of bed. Of course, you're asking yourself all the time what could have gone wrong. You haven't a clue. As you walk to the bathroom, you realize the pain is worse on the left side; you get an extra twinge there every time you take a step. Probably a muscular strain is what's causing your spasm.

When dealing with pain, looking for a pattern is always advisable. Begin by asking yourself standard questions: Have you ever experienced a similar pain? Can you associate unusual activities or positions with the occasions you have felt this pain or something like it? Maybe you reached under the car seat for a dropped coin or struggled to open an especially recalcitrant door. Have you gone rollerblading or horseback riding, carried heavy grocery bags to and fro, helped a neighbor clip a hedge?

Has a similar pain occurred after doing something you usually do or maintaining a position you're normally in, but this time you overdid it? Did you spend an extra hour in an uncomfortable chair because you couldn't put down the mystery you were reading? At the movies did you have to crane your neck and strain to the right to see around the giant in front of you?

Perhaps something has just begun. Believe it or not, the addition to your life of a new girlfriend or boyfriend could be the source of your backache. Or the reason may be less sublime: your desk at the office has just been replaced, let's say, or you're wearing new shoes with a significantly different heel.

Look for likely causes by repeating, one by one, any actions you think might have caused your pain. The responsible activity will reproduce the same pain. If you succeed in finding the problem this way, obviously you know what action to avoid.

Unfortunately, as hard and as cleverly as you may try, you can't always find the cause of your problem, sometimes because it has become chronic or has more than one cause. When pain persists, it can create intentional or unintentional adaptations. For example, you might favor one leg or sleep in a particular position. Chronic pain is complex, and it can be negatively affected by mood.

Since parts of the brain that are influenced by mood directly modify coordination and posture, it's worth thinking about your recent emotional state. You could say that characteristic stances represent pride, defiance, or the slump of depression. While some of these essential examples of body language can alleviate low back pain, others can cause it—by increasing the load on already tired muscles, thus overworking them and possibly pushing them into spasm.

Regardless of your success in finding the activity (or mood) that caused your pain, if it gets worse the second or third day[1] and then starts to get better, you've probably fallen victim to one of the many muscular or postural problems. If you can activate your pain through pressure or a specific movement, and if massaging that spot or lying in a warm bath seems to help, there's a high probability that your problem is musculoskeletal; in other words, it stems from spasm, strain, sprain, subluxation, or mild dislocation of muscles, ligaments, or bones. (I will explain these four conditions shortly.) Exquisite, off-the-charts pain is associated with fracture and indicates that you need an X ray.

When to Stretch, When to Rest

Musculoskeletal problems have only two basic mechanisms for producing pain. Either muscles have gone into spasm or you've suffered

[1]Add a day to this waiting period if you're between the ages of 45 and 50, add three days if you are 55 to 60, and so on.

a mishap related to movement. Treatment depends on the origin of your pain:

- For spasm—stretching is the primary answer, though the cure might cause more pain for the first few minutes.
- For strain, sprain, subluxation, and dislocation—rest, possibly with support, is the remedy. When you've suffered from problems related to movement, activity can actually further the process which caused the injury in the first place, causing more pain. Though rest helps you heal, it should not go on so long that it allows the joint capsule, tendon, or ligaments to stiffen and restrict your range of motion. Severe strain, sprain, subluxation, and dislocation may require medical treatment.
- Severe bruising may also need medical attention. Of course, if a trauma has caused only simple bruising, the pain will disappear by itself.

Spasm

All of a sudden the muscles in your back seem to take over and contract on their own. Spasm, this type of low back pain, may feel like a charley horse or a cramp, only more extreme. A charley horse occurs in a visible muscle, but you can't see the problem with lower back muscles when they are in spasm. In addition to being behind you and out of sight, these muscles are postural and not usually under your direct, conscious control.

The difference between a normal muscle contraction and a spasm is that a spasm is always intense and involuntary. A built-in "engineering defect" may be responsible. When a muscle clenches, no matter why, it's working. It needs an increased blood supply to provide oxygen and food, and to carry away the waste products of its own metabolism. But that very contraction makes it more difficult for the little blood vessels that run through the muscle to deliver nutrients and remove toxins. A local, temporary buildup of acid that the blood flow could not remove causes further tightness. Then we're off on the well-known vicious cycle: the spasm produces acids, and the acids increase spasm. This severe pain is often misunderstood by doctors and loved ones, who may suppose the cause of such intense discomfort to be ominous, but the good news is that it's not serious and need not be long-lasting.

What to Do   Stretching is the main cure for spasm. In addition to stretching, gentle massage along the length of the affected muscle, and not across it, is often useful. Warm baths and hot packs soothe the ache.

Spasm can last a moment or can hang on for a long time. If pain doesn't abate and you see a doctor or other health-care worker, you might ask for a prescription for ultrasound (see Chapter 11) to dilate muscular blood vessels, provide relief, and speed tissue repair. A physical therapist can help with assisted range of motion, or a physician can inject a painkiller. An injection of anesthetic interrupts the vicious cycle by temporarily paralyzing or at least relaxing the muscle and allowing blood circulation to return to normal. High- and low-voltage electric currents applied by a physical therapist can fatigue a muscle so that it has to relax, which also normalizes circulation. Each method involves intervening and stopping the vicious cycle.

Even before you have your pain under control, you should start thinking about prevention. Scrutinize your activities—the new bed you bought, the way you pick up the growing baby—and find out how you're inadvertently triggering the pain in your back.

Strain

Strain is just what it sounds like—damage due to the application of excessive force. The fibers that make up muscles, ligaments, tendons, joint coverings, or the joints themselves are pulled out of their normal alignment or formation. Strain, as described by physiatrist Renee Cailliet (in his book *Soft Tissue Pain and Disability*), can occur when:

- there is undue force on a normal structure (lifting an object that is too heavy);
- there is normal force on an abnormally frail joint, muscle, tendon, or ligament;
- there is normal stress on a normal but unprepared structure (a sedentary person who dances all night);
- you are performing an awkward weight-bearing activity (for example, putting a suitcase in an airplane's overhead compartment).

What to Do   Rest and relaxation allow the natural healing processes to occur. Nonsteroidal antiinflammatory medication can reduce pain and inflammation. Of course, recalling the event that caused the strain and avoiding it during the healing period will prevent reinjury.

Sprain

Strain turns into sprain when the fibers of muscles, tendons, ligaments, or joint capsules are pulled so forcibly that some of them actually tear (Figure 9). These usually heal by themselves with time, but not always. It's odd, but a sprain can be more serious and disabling than a fracture. For one thing, sprains heal slowly; for another, they tend to recur because of decreased blood supply to the muscle or structure when it is under chronic stress.

What to Do   A sprained ankle needs to be taped or given some other means of support. Air casts, Unna boots, or other types of braces are options. Rest, support, and nonsteroidal antiinflammatories also help.

When muscles, tendons, or ligaments in the spine are sprained, the answer is rest, ultrasound, massage, and then, as you start to improve, gentle range-of-motion exercises. Unfortunately, sometimes neither the victim nor the physician takes a sprain seriously enough to treat it.

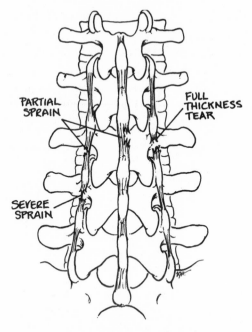

PARTIAL
SPRAIN

FULL
THICKNESS
TEAR

SEVERE
SPRAIN

Figure 9. A sprain is a tear in a ligament, shown here, or in a tendon.

Subluxation and Dislocation

When a joint experiences enough strain, there can be a mild change in the position of the bones. Subluxation refers to the situation when the surfaces inside a joint aren't in perfect spatial relationship with each other because one or both bones are slightly out of alignment. When there is subluxation, the joint is functional, though the bones aren't in their normal positions. Subluxation turns into dislocation when these surfaces are so far out of alignment they're unlikely to go back to normal on their own.

What to Do

Subluxation Manual medical manipulation is a fundamental part of chiropractic, and chiropractors are good at realigning bones. Osteopaths and physical therapists using manual medicine techniques are also effective.

Dislocation The pain of clearly evident dislocation is more severe in proportion to the derangement. This is not common, and is usually preceded by trauma or long, progressive degeneration. X rays are used for diagnosis. Since spinal stability is threatened by this serious condition, an orthopedist or neurosurgeon should be involved as soon as possible.

Self-Examination for Musculoskeletal Pain

If there is tenderness in your lumbar spine—that is, if you can produce pain by pressing with your fingers on your lower back—that's probably where the trouble is, and the muscles you're touching are the likely villains.

1. Put your thumbs against your spine, move them out two to three inches toward each side, and press. If this produces pain, the problem is in two muscles: the quatratus lumborum and the serratus inferior posterior (Figure 10). These muscles work to extend our backs, holding us up against the pull of gravity when we're leaning forward. They probably hurt now because of improper lifting.

2. Put your hands on your hips, and move your thumbs up gradually. If there's pain in the muscles at your side (the curving parts of the ribs), the problem could well have resulted from any of the following activities: moving abruptly from one side to the other, carrying a pail of water in one hand, twisting, parking a vehicle without power steering, cross-country skiing, or awkward repetitive movements.

3. Get a friend to press between the bones in your back or do it yourself. If this causes pain, you probably have strained or sprained ligaments. However, when pain occurs inside the spinal column it-

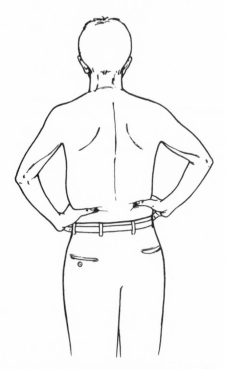

Figure 10. Thumb pressure should be applied a few inches away from the spine, midway between the last rib and the pelvis.

self, and doesn't increase with pressure, it could signal a more serious (not musculoskeletal) problem.

4. For pain in the buttocks, once again the diagnosis is at your fingertips. Generalized muscular pain in this area can result from too much running, arching of the back, pushing, or sitting. Sometimes the pain is in specific spots, as when the muscle gets so tight it pinches the sciatic nerve (see the section on piriformis syndrome in Chapter 9). Pain can also occur at the outsides of the buttocks near the hip joints, or near the bones you sit on. (See the discussion of bursitis below.)

Mimics of Musculoskeletal Pain

Range-of-motion difficulties and bursitis aren't exactly musculoskeletal problems. Nevertheless, these two conditions have many of the same symptoms and cures.

RANGE OF MOTION

There are normal, well-defined limits to how far a wrist or spine or any joint in the body will move. Tight muscles or a joint capsule that isn't working properly can reduce these limits, called range of motion. This often comes about after an injury or because of a sedentary lifestyle. Sometimes just one joint is affected when range of motion is decreased. When many joints in the back and elsewhere lose range of motion, the person has to adapt, and pain can be a consequence.

I saw an example of this in a twenty-five-year-old woman who had sprained her ankle severely six years before. Though her foot had been braced at the time and treated well, reduced range of motion now prevented her from bringing that foot up far enough when walking. The adaptation she had to make amounted to a gait irregularity that caused pain in her back.

What to Do   Though loss of range of motion isn't the same as muscle spasm, the answer to this problem is the same—stretching and strengthening the muscles. A combination of physical therapy with ultrasound and manual medicine is the right choice.

Osteoarthritis caused reduced range of motion in the neck of a patient who writes romance novels. She couldn't raise her head to see the computer screen. As for many others in the same boat, the answer to her problem lay in increasing the flexibility of the spine; training helped her to compensate with nearly unaffected vertebrae so she could continue turning out her bodice-ripping adventures.

Bursitis

The inflammation occurs because often repetitive trauma irritates the little fluid-filled pouches meant to isolate one structure from another and prevent irritation where the paths of muscles and bones cross. When these pouches get irritated they swell, causing further irritation in a vicious cycle. Like a subluxation or dislocation, pressing on the trouble spot hurts. Movement makes it worse. You may be able to identify the activity that produces the pain. (See Chapter 9.)

For example, one patient had a bursal problem below the knee, a common predicament with typical repercussions. Walking, which of course he couldn't avoid, made matters worse, causing him to favor the knee and producing back pain.

What to Do   You can't cure bursitis on your own. An injection of a combination of lidocaine and steroid almost always works for at least three months, allowing time for you to turn your attention to gait irregularities or treatment of joint problems that caused the bursitis in the first place.

What Musculoskeletal Pain Is Not

With musculoskeletal pain there is no tingling or numbness, no feelings of hot, cold, pins and needles, or anything else to suggest pain of neurological origins. You may find it painful and therefore undesirable to move, but you're not weak and you can move if you want to. Your legs are their normal color and temperature. You feel all right in general, and don't have any skin rashes, stomach upsets, or fever related to the painful feeling.

CHAPTER 6

Numbness

NOT FEELING WHAT *IS* THERE

I n the last two chapters we've discussed pain. Much as we don't
like pain, we need this sensation to alert us when something's
wrong. Producing pain is certainly one of the most important
functions of nervous systems throughout the animal kingdom. That's
why as many as 95 percent of our little nerve fibers are devoted to
the transmission of impulses that end up with this unpleasant but
often protective experience.

Numbness, strange sensations (paresthesias), and weakness are
fundamentally different from pain. They're manifestations of abnormal rather than normal nervous system activity. Nevertheless,
they too let us in on problems that need attention. We feel numbness
when nerve impulses don't travel, as they should, from the skin to the
brain. Paresthesias occur when "static" somewhere along a nerve's
pathway makes it suggest stimuli that don't exist in reality. And weakness results from signals not traveling properly from the brain to the
muscles, or from problems in the muscles themselves.

An understanding of pain depends on knowledge of the laws of
cause and effect: "once burnt, twice shy." To grasp the principles of

numbness, paraesthesia, and weakness you need information about the nervous system, how it functions, and how it can go awry. Familiarity with muscle function is also necessary for an understanding of weakness. Chapters 6 through 8 give insight into how problems in the nervous system produce these common and curious phenomena. Then, in Chapter 9, I will go over the way patterns of numbness, paresthesias, and weakness come together and characterize the different causes of back pain.

If you have back problems, you may also experience numbness (reduced or absent skin sensitivity) in other parts of your body, especially the legs and feet. This deserves serious attention. It always indicates nerve damage of some kind in the peripheral nervous system or in the central nervous system, that is, in the spine or brain.

Numbness occurs in the skin and the linings of body orifices, like the mouth and vagina. The same condition deep within the body, say in the liver, is called "insensate." There are degrees of numbness: At the far end of the spectrum is anesthesia, when you feel nothing, not the prod of a pin or a stone in your shoe. At the other end is reduced sensation, which can be close to imperceptible. Here's an example of the latter.

Recently a pediatric cardiologist whose children and mine go to the same school consulted me about his back pain and sciatica. In the past two years this physician has taken up jogging and is now preparing to run a marathon. Having gone through medical school, and having worked with a superb personal trainer, I thought that of all people this thirty-five-year-old man in his prime would be able to examine himself and report accurately on his symptoms. Yet during a short session in my office, we both received a surprise. A swath of numbness ran from his navel to mid-thigh. In all his pondering of his condition, in all the informal tests he had done on himself, this physician simply hadn't noticed a lack of feeling over a fairly large area of his body.

There's humor in the idea that a person can be numb to his or her own numbness, but diminished or absent feeling is no laughing matter. It's a warning flag that can help lead to diagnosis and treatment of back pain. My friend the pediatric cardiologist would have known he had a nerve-root injury if he'd been as astute when observing himself as he is with his patients, and he could have begun treatment several months sooner.

A person's perception of numbness is a symptom. I listen carefully to subjective reports of this symptom, note it in a patient's history, and use it in my thinking about a case. In addition, numbness can be tested objectively, and the results of those tests are signs that also point toward a diagnosis.

Though it often accompanies pain, numbness might not seem as "important." But frequently numbness is a *more* reliable guide than pain for a doctor trying to make a diagnosis. The reason for this, as I've said before, is that pain is subjective. It can change in character, can be difficult to locate precisely, and can radiate. When you feel pain in one place, you might compensate in another, creating a "red herring" of a symptom. On the other hand, numbness is actual and objective, and testing for it shouldn't be restricted only to physicians. As the patient and the person experiencing the symptoms, you can find out exactly where and to what extent your sensitivity is diminished.

Self-Examination

LIGHT TOUCH

Simple Pin Test   Doctors use a simple pin test to determine objectively whether a person feels pain or experiences any sensation. This measure is valid whether the patient's condition is as serious as a coma or as mild as a bruise. A set of thin wands, the Semmes-Weinstein filaments, have calibrated stiffness to measure numbness exactly. The results of this test are objective—assuming the patient is really trying to report accurately, without minimizing or maximizing.

There's no reason you can't do what professionals do and test yourself for numbness. Use a sharp pencil, which has the advantage of marking exactly the point you have just touched. Another handy tool for self-examination is a toothpick. Practice a little so that taps on your skin are uniform in strength. With your attention focused, and being careful not to damage your skin, you will be able to determine for yourself the degree of your own sensation, whether it is reduced, normal, or enhanced.

Spacing   Another objective measure is how far apart two points have to be before you perceive them as two separate points. Hold two pins between thumb and index finger to keep them at a fixed distance; test first a normal skin area and then an affected region to compare and discover where the two points are distinct. You can measure the distance between them with a ruler. On abnormal skin, pins will be farther apart.

HOT AND COLD

When you're numb, you may have much less awareness of the feelings of hot or cold. Begin with a part of your body you're sure is experiencing normal sensation. Using an ice cube and a warm washcloth, look for a pattern of numbness by comparing how vividly you sense the temperature in symmetrical locations (that is, in the same places on the left and right sides of your body). If the right and left sides don't match, the exact area that differs (the outside of the ankle, for example) will give you a clue as to the location of the problem. Generally (but not always), the bigger the area that is affected, the higher in the body the origin is. Most of the rest of this chapter is devoted to this topic.

REFLEXES

Obviously, numbness can reduce or obliterate reflexes. Chapter 8 will give a full description of reflex testing. For the moment, bear in mind that reflexes require a sensory input such as a tap or a nudge that the nervous system must register before making the body respond.

The results of reflex tests determine whether the problem originates in the brain, the spinal cord, or the peripheral nerves.

Most doctors test reflexes, but few do sensation (numbness) testing. It's amazing to me that doctors have become so hard pressed as to leave this out of routine testing. However, if you do a test yourself and report abnormalities, your physician should certainly take you seriously.

Locating the Problem

One of the marvels of neuroanatomy is that on our skin there are definite lines of demarcation (with a little overlap) between the territory of one nerve and another. For the most part these boundaries are quite exact and vary little from individual to individual. By testing areas of the skin for numbness, a physician can locate and identify particular groups of distressed nerve fibers. That narrows the field of investigation to some point along the course of those nerve fibers.

An example is the median nerve, which carries sensation from the middle of your ring finger and over the palm to and including the thumb. The other side of your hand—the little finger to the midline of the ring finger—is ruled by the ulnar nerve. Using simple pin testing on the skin on the right and left sides of your ring fingertip, you and your doctor can diagnose and distinguish between a problem in the median nerve and the ulnar nerve.

Basic Neuroanatomy

Before discussing how exact areas of numbness relate to spinal nerve-root problems, I want to explain that nerve fibers originate in the brain, run down the spinal cord, and branch out from there until they reach their preordained, specific regions in the body. These fibers

AREAS SERVED BY SPINAL-NERVE ROOTS

The nerve root at L1 serves the groin.

L2 relates to the front of the thigh.

L3 and L4 connect to the knee, the inside of the calf, and the instep.

The big toe and inside arch of the foot connect to L5.

S1 supplies sensation to the little-toe side of the foot.

S2 serves the back of the calf.

There is a thin region up the back of the leg to the buttocks that receives ennervation from S3.

The ring around the anus and the genital regions is served by S2 to S4.

leave the spine between each pair of vertebrae in bundles called nerve roots. The fibers from different nerve roots combine to form individual nerves, for example, the sciatic nerve.

LARGE PERIPHERAL NERVES

There are only two large nerves in each leg. Many of the fibers from L4 through S3 travel together after they combine in the lumbosacral plexus to form the sciatic nerve. The sciatic nerve itself divides above the knee to form the posterior tibial nerve (which serves the back of the calf and the sole of the foot) and the peroneal nerve (which serves the skin on the outside of the calf and top of the foot). The other large nerve is called the femoral nerve. This comes out of the plexus with fibers from L2, L3, and L4 and serves the inside of the calf and the instep. One large, purely sensory nerve—the femoral cutaneous— brings feeling to a point below the knee.

Incredibly, you yourself can go a long way toward determining whether the pain you feel in your back is due to root involvement at one or more of those levels just by noting the signs and symptoms associated with your numbness, paresthesias, and/or weakness and where these signs and symptoms coincide. See Chapter 9. In the meantime you can learn more about your numbness by reading on.

Peripheral Nervous System

The sensory parts of the peripheral nervous system (PNS) consist of the end organs that are the "outskirts" of the nervous system, at the frontier between the person and the outside environment. These tiny nerve endings lie in the skin and just below it, and they take various shapes. Some, which look like little coils, register pressure. Some are spidery-looking free nerve endings that report an overabundance of any stimulus. Others look like balls with sticks coming out and sense vibrations. And still others are tubular end organs that respond when lightly compressed. All of these report to the central nervous system. If a flame touches your fingertip, a combination of fibers will send the burning sensation to your brain. When those receptor coils, tubes, and balls don't function, the finger will burn but you will feel nothing. If the same combination of nerve fibers is compressed in the spine, your brain will receive no signals, even if the nerve endings on the skin of your fingertip are functioning perfectly. How much attention the central nervous system pays to reports from its distant outposts depends on the conduction of nerve fibers that give the report (see Figure 11 on page 123).

There is not a one-to-one correspondence of nerve fibers to sensations. Instead, nerve fibers are constantly sending a regularly timed rhythm of signals to the brain. This background pattern is like a silent drum tattoo, which serves as assurance that everything is all right. When this complex, "all is well" rhythm stops or changes, the central nervous system then fixes its attention on the pathways between the brain and the source.

WELL-KNOWN CAUSES OF PNS NUMBNESS

Compressed or injured nerves, generalized systemic conditions, and circulatory problems are the most common causes of numbness originating in the peripheral nervous system.

Pinched Nerves   Nerves are often entrapped (pinched or compressed) as they leave the spine, in the buttock, and just below the knee.

Systemic Conditions   Diabetes is the most common cause of numbness. Too much sugar in a person's blood stream is toxic to nerve cells, whose structure and function deteriorate and which soon begin to die out. At that time, generalized numbness sets in, usually in the parts of the body most distant from the central nervous system—the lower legs and feet. Kidney disease and thyroid abnormalities, also, can kill some nerve fibers and slow down the conduction of others. This causes many signals to reach the brain later than would be normal. The disruption of the usual pattern of signals is more severe the farther those signals have to travel. These conditions are called neuropathies.

Toxic exposure, drugs, or autoimmune or other systemic problems can also result in neuropathies. Nerve conduction is slowed, which drastically reduces sensation, generally beginning in both the feet and lower legs. Though some neuropathies can be diagnosed and treated, others are difficult to identify and cure.

Neuropathies often affect motor as well as sensory nerves. Back pain is associated with neuropathies because weakness in the ankles and feet changes the way people walk and stand, abnormally stressing the back. In most neuropathies, the farther away from the brain, the more pronounced the numbness. The pattern is usually the same in both legs and feet. The higher on the leg, the less the numbness. There are no sharp boundaries between normal and numb areas. In exceptional circumstances a single nerve can be involved, but usually this is not associated with back pain.

Circulatory Difficulties   Your legs "fall asleep" or become numb when arterial circulation is hampered to the extent that nerves aren't getting enough nourishment to function well. The cure is to get the blood circulating again by changing position and moving around. Everyone's feet fall asleep sometimes. This phenomenon isn't associated with low back pain. If you feel no pain in your calves when walking a few blocks, it's doubtful that you have an arterial circulatory problem. If you do regularly feel pain after walking relatively short distances, see your doctor. Your problem could be connected with back pain in a condition called Le Riche syndrome, where narrow blood vessels in the area of the buttocks reduce blood flow, producing pain in the back and buttocks and numbness in the feet. But numbness and low back pain aren't always related.

A portly patient in his late fifties complained of intermittent but extreme numbness in his right foot. He also had back pain. While he sat in my office discussing when to schedule diagnostic tests, I noticed that he had crossed his left leg over his right. I observed him as he remained in the same position for more than fifteen minutes. As our conversation ended, I speculated out loud that when he stood up his right foot would be numb. I was correct. The reason was that the weight of one leg on the other was putting enough pressure on the peroneal nerve to affect its sensory fibers. The condition this gentleman had is called peroneal palsy. His great weight caused his numbness and contributed to his low back pain, but otherwise his symptoms were unrelated.

Spinal Cord

There are two types of nerve tissue in the spine. One is nerve cell bodies, which connect with each other to limit reflexes and make postural responses. These have the authority to give muscles orders to shift your body when, for example, you've been in one position for too long. They don't need to consult the brain, nor do they wait for orders to activate.

The second type consists of the long nerve fibers themselves that travel from the spine to everywhere throughout the body, reaching from the skin and muscles to the brain. Most of the nerve cell bodies that register reports from the lower back and legs are located in the lower thoracic spine and below.

Progressive damage to the spinal cord often shows up in the form of changes in sensation before pain and weakness arise. Nerve rootlets in the lumbar spine are arranged like targets, with sensory fibers on the outside and motor fibers on the inside. That's why pain and numbness precede muscle weakness (Figure 11).

Sensory fibers and motor fibers leave the spine separately, so an injury right at the point of departure might not impair motor activities but could significantly affect sensation. An interruption in the reports of sensation fibers can produce not only feelings of numbness but also hot and cold, pressure, movement, and muscle tightness.

WELL-KNOWN SPINAL CAUSES OF NUMBNESS

Radiculopathy   A pinched nerve due to herniated disk, for example, can cause an interruption in the function of sensory nerve fibers and changes in feeling.

Stenosis   Narrowness can squeeze sensory nerve fibers inside the spinal canal, causing loss of sensation. The degree of numbness can vary from next to nothing to complete anesthesia, but *where* it occurs

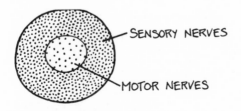

Figure 11. A cross section of a nerve rootlet.

is telling. It will be at multiple root levels and it may be on both sides of the body.

Multiple Sclerosis and Stroke   The disease processes of multiple sclerosis (MS) and stroke can take place in the spinal cord as well as in the brain, affecting sensation and also motor functions. MS is often described as whimsical because numbness can change from one place to another without warning or explanation.

Brain

Most back pain doesn't originate in the brain. That part of us, however, plays an important role in numbness.

In the 1950s, Dr. Robert Penfield gathered a tremendous amount of information about sensory nerves by experimenting on patients while doing brain surgery, often to save their lives. The patients were awake during the operations, and when the doctor stimulated given points in their brains, they would feel as though something was being done to them, such as someone squeezing a finger, or as though they were doing something, like running. The good doctor found that specific parts of the body were represented in an order resembling the body itself in the portion of the brain allotted to receiving sensory stimuli: the sensory homunculus (Figure 12).

In ancient times, people believed each sperm contained a tiny man or woman called "the humunculus," who eventually was born and grew to adulthood. Of course, that isn't true. But in the brain there are actually two structures that represent the entire human body. The motor humunculus (also called the motor strip) is a band of nerve cells stretching from the top of the brain toward each ear. The motor strip serves as the command center for impulses that move fingers, feet, and other parts of the body. Parallel to the motor strip and just behind it is the sensory humunculus, or sensory strip. The sensory strip tells you whether you're plunging your toe into ice water,

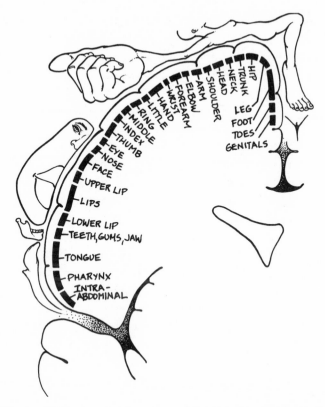

Figure 12. The sensory homunculus in the brain contains groups of cells representing all the different parts of the body. Any activation of those cells will be perceived as coming from that part of the body even if it isn't coming from there. For example, nerve fibers from your ankle may be irritated at L5 as they travel up your spine to the brain. Though the pain is caused in your back, you will feel it in your ankle.

experiencing numbness, or tasting a pear poached in rum. It's that group of cells that concerns us now.

The brain structure that receives sensory input has a miraculously specialized design. All the cells that register reports from the thumb, for instance, are concentrated in one place. All the cells that get information from the side of the face are in another place; from a specific area in the back in still another, and so on. Injury to those brain cells can prevent perception of a specific location or interrupt the reports of sensation, resulting in numbness in that part of the body.

DIAGNOSTIC TESTING

When you have a loss of sensation due to a problem with a particular nerve, the trouble can be anywhere along the course of that nerve, from the bottom of the little toe to the sensory strip in the brain. Neurologists and physiatrists use SSEPs (somatosensory evoked potentials) to find the exact location of the difficulty.

Mild electrical stimuli are applied to parts of the body and picked up by electrodes placed on the scalp over the responsive part of the brain. Doctors measure the size, shape, and timing of the nervous impulses reaching the brain and generally can locate the injury with accuracy. For instance, if stimulation at the ankle gives abnormal responses in the brain but nervous impulses from the knee to the appropriate part of the cerebrum are normal, the problem lies between the knee and ankle.

WELL-KNOWN CEREBRAL CAUSES OF NUMBNESS

Stroke   Usually stroke involves the arm, leg, trunk, or face on one side only. A stroke on the right side of the cortex often brings numbness to the left side of the body in a pattern all its own. If the stroke occurred in the part of the sensory homunculus that registers signals from the outside of the leg, that's where the patient will have the numbness, often accompanied by weakness, lack of coordination, and heightened reflexes. A stroke in the front of the brain usually involves legs more than arms. A blood clot the middle of the brain affects the arms and face. These specific areas and patterns are rarely associated with low back pain.

Seizures   Uncontrollable movements of seizures can bring about back pain but that's not all. A tumor that causes seizures, personality and memory difficulties, and pain in the face, as well as arms and legs, can also cause difficulties with movement and subsequent back pain.

Congenital Abnormalities   If at birth there are malformations of the veins or arteries in the head, there could be episodes where numbness comes and goes. This is often hereditary, and again, patterns are different from those related to low back pain.

Concussion   Injury to the head often results in injury to the spine as well. A blow to the head can cause concussion and result in numbness in the face. If an athlete suffers from a second concussion shortly after the first, the results are often catastrophic.

Generalized Conditions   Multiple sclerosis (MS), for example, can involve more than one limb in various ways (such as tingling combined with numbness) and can also vary in intensity. Back pain is sometimes an initial symptom.

Psychological Upsets   It's uncommon today, but numbness is sometimes attributed to an emotional problem, specifically hysteria. It's accompanied by what's called "la belle indifference," which gives the patient a good-natured attitude about the inability to feel. There's no known physiological cause for this, so it's often used as a diagnosis of last resort.

A more common psychological cause of numbness is hyperventilation brought about by high anxiety. Fast breathing brings too much oxygen and too little carbon dioxide to the circulating blood, causing numbness and tingling of hands, feet, and often around the mouth. This frightening condition, which can be brought on by extremely severe back pain, quickly disappears when a change in situation or physical position produces a difference in breathing pattern.

———

Most of us would prefer numbness to pain, but actually the two symptoms may come from the same cause—something adversely affecting the nervous system. In the case of pain, the nervous system may just be reliably reporting danger signs. Numbness may be more serious than pain because the nervous system may be out of commission, unable to issue warning signals. Sometimes, however, the nervous system falls prey to an intermediate state and is able to report, but inaccurately. Paresthesias, the subject of the next chapter, are a prime example of this.

CHAPTER 7

Paresthesias

FEELING WHAT *ISN'T* THERE

Paresthesias are sensations you feel for no apparent reason. Just as anesthesia (numbness) is not feeling what *is* there, paresthesia is feeling things that *aren't* there. These feelings are almost always located on the skin. You may experience burning or tingling on one calf, though nothing is touching it. The sensation of shocks, pins and needles, ants crawling, or tightness of the skin are other common paresthesias. These aren't imagination, because the feeling is real. People who suffer from strange sensations consider them annoying, distracting, and uncomfortable, but they don't always know why they have them.

An elderly gentleman came to me with what he thought was a problem in his feet. "Maybe my shoes are pinching something," he said. "Please look at them and see where they need fixing. They make my feet tingle when I put them on, and they make my feet tingle when I take them off and lie down. It's got to be the shoes, because I felt fine when I was sitting around the pool in Palm Springs last month."

The man's shoes were practically new. His feet showed no abnormalities. I questioned him about whether he experienced tingling when he took his daily walks. He didn't think so. Did his back ache? Yes. With the addition of his final answer about backache, I had enough information to check for spinal stenosis (see Figure 4 on page 72), which I found.

Although this patient had back pain, it is possible to have strange sensations with or without backache. Every time these unusual feelings occur with back pain, however, they are crucial diagnostic clues.

Similarities between Numbness and Paresthesias

We're all built more or less alike, and that includes our nerves. Specific nerves are made up of motor and sensory fibers that each serve the same regions of every person's body. The motor fibers stimulate the muscles they control when a person decides it's time to move. Sensory fibers serve exact, identifiable skin areas called dermatomes (Figure 13). When there is an injury at a nerve root, paresthesias may occur in these dermatomes. (See Figure 15 on page 152.)

Like numbness, paresthesias have their origins in the brain, spinal cord, or peripheral nervous system. In general, they have the same causes as numbness, and like numbness they're usually attributable to a neurological cause (see Chapter 6). Because they're sensations, with few exceptions these feelings occur in the distribution of affected nerves, the way numbness does. For example, spinal cord injury of the left fifth lumbar nerve root can produce numbness in the big toe and inner part of the foot, coupled with tingling and other paresthesias in the same places.

Compression or pinching of a peripheral nerve, either in the spinal canal at the root level, in the plexuses (junctures) where spinal nerve roots meet and regroup, in the buttock or in the leg can produce paresthesias. In other words, nerve fibers serving a particular area must be able to send impulses all the way to the brain to bring our usual sensations to consciousnesses.

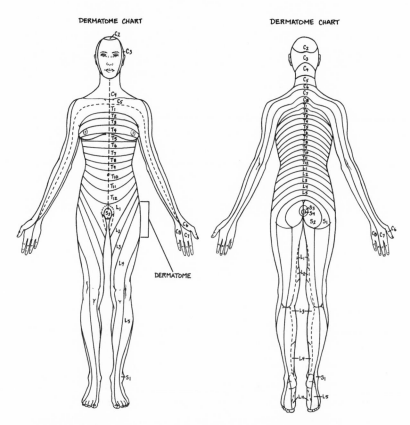

Figure 13. There is an exact relationship between the cause of a neurological symptom and where you feel it. For example, tingling in the dermatome at the inside of the kneecap is due to problems at L3.

Paresthesias occur when disruption in this transmission is severe enough to alter the normal pattern of communication to our cerebral cortex but mild enough to allow most nerve impulses to get through. The disruption can occur anywhere along the way. When coupled with low back pain or sciatica, the site of the disturbance is usually in the buttocks, pelvis, or spine.

Differences between Numbness and Paresthesias

While there are many similarities between numbness and paresthesias, there are also differences. For one thing, strange sensations have no observable cause. Nor are there any objective tests for paresthesias. The way to test for numbness is by pressing a given skin area with the point of a pin. An equal amount of pressure will produce more (or less) sensation, depending on the patient's condition. There's a difference with paresthesias. When it comes to these strange sensations, you can't isolate any one spot on the skin by using pressure, a thermometer, or other methods. The sensations occur without anything happening in places where it seems something must be happening. Nothing is "there."

An example of the objective difference between paresthesias and numbness is that numbness exists and can be demonstrated in a sleeping patient. A patient can be pricked with a pin, or receive an electric shock, and he or she will sleep on; an unconscious person doesn't feel paresthesias.

However, paresthesias are sometimes reproducible. If you have a herniated disk, bending forward can cause sciatica or weakness when you point your toes. By performing the same movements, you might recreate tingling on the side of the leg. This provides a substantial clue as to its cause. You can look up the pattern of involvement on the skin for paresthesias by using the Nerve-Root Symptoms Chart (see Figure 15 on page 152) to locate the possible origin of the problem more precisely.

As said before, in general, the causes of paresthesias are the same as the causes of numbness. Paresthesias occur when nerve fibers are affected and functioning erratically. Numbness occurs when those same nerve fibers aren't functioning at all. Still, there are a few things that will cause one and not the other.

Phantom Pain and Phantom Sensation

An amputee might feel as if someone were twisting or crushing the foot or toes, particularly the big toe or ankle. These unpleasant experiences are known as phantom pain. This phenomenon, though not extremely common, is interesting and important.

In a person who's healthy and whole, the nervous system is constantly transmitting a pattern of impulses that go along the spinal cord to various parts of the brain. This continuous, normal pattern assures us that everything is all right. When you lose a limb, however, the situation changes. The missing part of the body can no longer generate its pattern. When the brain isn't receiving impulses from the lost limb anymore, it may substitute input from elsewhere or nerve cells may spontaneously discharge, creating the image of some sensation. These feelings are sometimes painful, and they sometimes simulate what the person felt when losing the limb.

Still, there is a cure for phantom pain. Standard treatment involves presenting the amputee with simple, verifiable sensory stimulation, like having the individual watch himself rub a piece of soft leather on the stump of a leg. The patient often begins to experience fewer painful sensations, and has feelings that are more connected with what is actually happening. This successful therapeutic technique, called sensory reintegration, when carried into daily life in connection with activities like walking or getting up from a chair, gradually helps eradicate pain.

Amputees also experience another phenomenon, called phantom sensation, which is common or even normal for these patients. In the appropriate context these sensations—for example, a thigh pressing against the sofa cushion or a breeze on one's leg—would be normal. Of course, these feelings aren't "normal" when the leg is absent. But they are considered phantom sensations rather than paresthesias because they aren't unpleasant. The feelings include hot and cold, light pressure, and the sense of moving or having the limb moved. As with phantom pain, phantom sensations often lessen with sensory reintegration.

However, people in possession of all their limbs also frequently fall victim to "phantom sensations." If you have back pain and one of your nerves isn't sending proper signals to your brain, you may experience all kinds of unusual feelings. This is the result of an alteration in normal patterns of nerve discharge and conduction, not something happening in the "affected" part of the body, such as the foot where the person feels the tingling. This kind of interference in normal patterning has sent millions of people to doctors for diagnosis. You should understand that the disruption not only causes paresthesias; it often goes along with sciatica or low back pain. The feeling is in the foot or leg, but the cause is in the back, far away.

Paresthesias and the Back

The location of strange sensations in the lower body almost always shows the way to a specific affected nerve root in the back. Paresthesias are analogous to the knockings in the engine of a car. You hear them, you know something is wrong, but in themselves they're not always motivation to go to the repair shop. If the knockings in the car engine get faster when you step on the accelerator and are accompanied by black smoke rising from the hood, you know you've got a problem. Given the car's signs and symptoms the repair person can probably make an educated guess about the cause of the smoke. In the same way, if you have paresthesias in the inner calf and pain going down the back of your leg, such paresthesias give a powerful direction to your investigation of the cause of the pain.

Here are some examples of locations of strange sensations and the corresponding affected nerve roots in the back:

• Strange sensations in the knee indicate a problem with the nerve at L3.
• Unusual feelings at the inner calf and ankle point to the nerve root at L4.

- If the outside of the foot is affected, the nerve root responsible is S1.
- The bottom of the foot sends signals to the nerve roots at L5 and S1.
- The region from the leg to rectal or genital regions is served by nerves going to S3 and S4.

Unusual Causes of Paresthesias

Both paresthesias and numbness can arise from a generalized condition that in unusual cases originates in the spinal cord. The strong outer covering of the whole central nervous system out to and including nerve roots is called the dura mater. When there is pressure against the dura mater for any reason, bafflingly diverse paresthesias may arise. For example, there may be tingling in one leg that moves all of a sudden to the other leg and then to the outside of the calf. These sensations can vary widely.

This condition is more serious if there's enough pressure so that the nerves themselves are involved, but in those cases the paresthesias localize and are easier to use in arriving at a diagnosis. When the pressure is even greater and the nerve conduction more seriously impaired, paresthesias give way to localized numbness. This numbness, when sufficiently severe, can turn into paresthesias again. Then it's like phantom pain.

Another condition, called allodynia, is a curious dysfunction of the nervous system. In these cases a normally innocuous stimulus, like the bed sheet touching your leg, is perceived as painful. Like numbness, it take some stimulation to be aware of this unpleasant sensation, and like paresthesia you feel something unrelated to what is happening. Allodynia is a consequence of burn, stroke, and reflex sympathetic dystrophy (injury in one part of the body causing the autonomic nervous system to produce painful symptoms elsewhere).

CHAPTER 8

Weakness

LOSING WHAT WAS THERE

N umbness and paresthesias have entirely neurological causes, but weakness (if it can't be traced to a systemic condition like diabetes) can come from either a nerve or muscle problem. Just as anesthesia is the extreme of numbness, paralysis is what occurs at the outer limit of weakness. In this chapter I'll discuss the many reasons people experience weakness related to low back pain. However, when all is said and done, it's wise to remember that the most usual cause of overall symmetrical weakness (equal weakness on the right and left in both arms and legs) is inactivity. Of course, weakness can also occur in only one place or on one side.

Muscle Weakness Resulting from Adaptation

If you isolate a finger in a cardboard tube for an hour or two and then stimulate that digit with heat, for example, it will be more sensitive than it was before. That's because protecting the finger from the outside world, "starving" it for stimulation, makes it more responsive.

The opposite is true of muscles. Stop using a muscle and very little time will pass before that muscle (and the limb it moves) will grow weaker. The weakness occurs and progresses rapidly toward atrophy, though the neurological connections are as perfect as they were in the finger. When it comes to any muscle, there is great truth in the saying "use it or lose it."

Muscles constitute the biggest system in our bodies; they make up literally as much as half of an individual. When you think about how much of us our muscles are, it's not surprising how frequently something goes wrong. In the vast majority of cases where weakness accompanies low back pain, the cause is muscular. There are various reasons muscular weakness comes about. Nearly invariably they are associated with the way we live our daily lives.

Posture, gait, step size, amount of arm swing when walking—all will affect literally scores of muscles in the middle and lower back. Even a minor injury like a sprain or strain of the gastrocnemius (the largest muscle in the calf), for example, can force an individual to adapt in many ways when walking. Both big and small adjustments to weakness of an injured muscle may have a domino effect, quickly producing considerable pain in the back. These adaptations take place silently and rapidly: one day everything's all right, and the next day the individual is in big trouble. "It happened so fast it must have been a nerve," one patient said. Not true. It seemed sudden, but it was the end result of a natural, unnoticed process through this patient's body, like all our bodies, adapted to its current conditions, reallocating force and function until the pain appeared.

A forty-two-year-old advertising executive and mother of two came to me complaining of severe, almost crippling back pain. "It's on the left just above the waist, in my back," she said. She felt stabbed with every step. This charming, sophisticated world traveler worked out regularly in a high-tech gym. Her stressful lifestyle didn't faze her. She looked ten years younger than she was, and aside from her back pain she felt fine—except for one thing. "It's got to be neurological," she told me, pointing to her thigh. "Look how this thigh has shrunk."

It was true. The left thigh was noticeably smaller, and it had happened in only three weeks. Because of isolated weakness in straightening her knee, her conclusion sounded right to me, but of course, I had to confirm her opinion. On the contrary, elaborate diagnostic testing turned up no nerve damage of any kind.

So I had to look further. Eventually we discovered that degenerative joint disease was the culprit. Because of an unnoticed leg-length discrepancy, osteoarthritis had started earlier for this lady than it does in most cases and had become rather severe in that leg. Her brain and spinal cord inhibited the quadriceps muscle (which straightens the knee joint), starting atrophy. Without realizing it she had devised a way of walking that made less use of the joint and muscle, and she continued to adapt until her backache gave her another sign. Ironically my patient barely remembered the original, mild pain in her hip that signaled the beginning of her trouble.

Involuntary adaptation to osteoarthritis in the knee joint occurred completely outside my patient's awareness. Without her consent, her nerves had changed their readiness to fire off and make muscles contract, because of the pain. The less the thigh muscles contracted, the weaker they became. This lack of strength caused her to swing the right leg around when walking, putting a lot of strain on her left lower back. The back muscles had to support the unergonomic swinging of the leg, resulting in overwork and painful spasm. The abnormal gait became more and more exaggerated, finally causing the severe symptoms that brought her to me.

This woman's story is actually quite common. Sometimes the patient is puzzled to hear the doctor say, "If you want to cure your low back pain, we'd better focus on the problem with your knee." Yet with regularity, physicians can diagnose the cause of back pain as a patient walks into the office.

My teacher, Dr. Edward Delagi, worked on a rehabilitation ward during World War II and saw firsthand how quickly the human body and mind adapt to new situations. A young soldier had suffered grave injuries when hit by shrapnel during battle. He had been recovering for quite some time when he was brought in for a surgical attempt to correct a problem that was relatively minor compared to his others: destruction of muscles had made the patient unable to raise his wrist. The surgery involved transplanting a healthy muscle and giving it that function.

While the operation was going on, Dr. Delagi studied the records and developed a plan to help the patient accommodate to his injury and improve his ability to move. An hour or two after the soldier recovered consciousness, Dr. Delagi had it all worked out and was ready to deliver his advice. "Nerves and muscles can be adapted to correct deficiencies . . ." he began.

"Yes, sir. Now I can do this," the patient replied with a smile. He raised his wrist effortlessly.

What struck Dr. Delagi was not only that the operation had been successful but that the patient's brain had acted so quickly to restore and orchestrate complex movements he hadn't been able to perform for many months.

The brain makes mystifyingly smooth adaptations to weakness and injury. If there are neurological problems in the back and a pattern of weakness, or weakness and numbness, it's often easy to arrive at a neurological diagnosis and treatment options. What's much more common but harder to figure out is how the repercussions of muscle weakness cause back pain.

Inactivity

By far the most common source of muscle weakness is inactivity. It occurs with people who sit all day, working hard but not using their muscles. Older people with modest activity levels also often experience this type of generalized weakness. You know that's your problem if the effort required to perform normal daily tasks, like wriggling into a slightly tight piece of clothing, leaves you breathless. This generalized deconditioning (a fall from peak performance levels) is characterized by symmetrical weakness.

Some signs and symptoms of muscle weakness due to inactivity and related to low back pain include:

• Propensity for Injury   A task like typing a twenty-page paper may not have been painful in the past but can cause back pain in a deconditioned person, because it requires unaccustomed postures and positions.

• Muscle Soreness   Doing something that doesn't seem strenuous can strain or sprain weak muscles, which are often in the back.

• Reduced Reflexes   Weakened muscles don't have the power to swing a limb very far.

Specific Muscle Weakness and Low Back Pain

Weakness can occur in the upper arms of person who rarely raises arms above head, or in the feet of someone who has needed leg casts, for instance, and who for some time hasn't used the plantar muscles in the feet for balance. These and similar situations can result in back pain. They require other, sometimes distant and mechanically disadvantaged muscles to perform unaccustomed tasks. For example, stabilizing your toes with the muscles in your foot is easy. Doing the same thing using muscles in the hip takes much more effort.

Specific weakness of the extensor muscles that help arch the back gets many people into trouble. It may develop from habitually sitting in chairs that provide too much support, from slouching, from reading propped up in bed, or from bending over for long periods of time.

The reason for this is that muscles are like magnets. The more the fibers overlap, the stronger the pull between them. When you slouch, you're stretching muscles quite a bit, pulling them so that they don't overlap as much and making them weaker.

Miscellaneous Causes of Muscle Weakness

Myopathy

Just like dermatitis, which affects the skin, and neuropathy, which affects the nerves, myopathy is a systemic condition that attacks muscle tissue, usually all over the body. These illnesses single out and weaken muscles. The various types of myopathy can come from diabetes and other endocrine abnormalities, from infections, and from autoimmune, toxic, and hereditary causes.

Most myopathies tend to show up first in muscles close to the trunk: the pectoralis muscles in the upper extremities and the iliopsoas muscles at the thigh. Because they move whole limbs, these muscles require more strength to do their work properly than muscles farther away on the arm or leg. If you have a myopathy, you'll notice weakness when walking up stairs. Your knees may involuntarily buckle at times, or jars may be harder to open. See your doctor. Good tests are available for diagnosing myopathies.

Osteoarthritis and Osteoporosis

These diseases of aging cause joint derangement and vertebral fractures, respectively. Nerve responses to these painful conditions weaken muscles (see Chapter 9).

Surgery

When a surgeon has to cut through muscles, they become weakened. Scar tissue doesn't contract, and local neurological connections are often severed. For example, one cosmetic surgery to repair a breast after mastectomy (transposition of the rectus abdominus muscle, or

TRAM) involves moving that muscle upward, which simultaneously weakens the anterior abdominal wall and makes the patient vulnerable to back pain.

Reflexes

A reflex involves sensation as well as muscle response. When you examine your reflexes, you are testing the sensory nerves; problems with these account for pain, strange sensations, and numbness, as already described in Chapters 6 and 7. You are also testing your motor nerves, which give strength, coordination, and control. Normal reflexes imply that the muscles are normal too, so coming up with normal reflexes is a great relief.

A reflex produces an involuntary response to stimulation (usually a light tap applied to a tendon). This is called a reflex arc. All reflex arcs involve sensory nerves that transmit an impulse, such as the impact on the tendon, to the spinal cord. There motor cells take over and contract a given muscle, for example, making the ankle flex.

The physiological function of reflexes is to protect muscles against weakness caused by overstretching. Tapping a tendon rapidly stretches the attached muscle. The reflex immediately contracts the muscle to its length of greatest strength.

There are reflexes all over the body. Some—a blink is an example—work without any physical contact. The knee and Achilles tendon reflexes are by far the most important for diagnosing the origins of back pain. These reflex arcs activate L2 through L4 (the knee reflex) and L5-S1 (the Achilles tendon reflex). (In the latter, when the tendon is tapped, the ankle flexes. Tapping the tendon stretches the muscle, sending "stretch sensations" to the spinal cord. This directly stimulates spinal-cord motor fibers, which make the muscle contract.) Most neurological back pain is caused by problems in the spine at L3 to L5 and at L5-S1.

The central nervous system controls reflexes, and sometimes produces an enhanced or unusually vigorous reflex that is abnormal, but we'll get to that discussion later in this chapter.

WELL-KNOWN REASONS FOR REDUCED OR ABSENT REFLEXES

When a reflex is weak or absent, any link in the chain may be at fault. Here are the four possibilities:

1. Neuropathy or other nerve damage impairs nerve impulse transmission.
2. Nerve entrapment or another mechanical problem interferes with motor or sensory impulses at a specific point.
3. There is a problem with the connection between nerves in the spine or between nerve and muscle. This connection is called a synapse.
4. There is muscle weakness.

Extreme muscle weakness all by itself can produce feeble reflex responses where there's nothing at all wrong with the nerves. You don't need reflex testing to know you have this situation. You will have dramatic loss of motor strength and be too weak to walk, for example, or to tap your feet to music. This rule also applies to reflexes that are diminished on one side only, as was the case with the patient with the arthritic knee. On the other hand, if you have normal muscle strength, right-sided sciatica, and reduced right Achilles tendon reflex, that's a sign of a problem with your L5-S1 nerve root, and sensation at the outside of your foot may be impaired.

REFLEX SELF-EXAMINATION

Knee   Sit comfortably in a straight-backed, unupholstered chair. Cross your legs. Make a fist. Tap the tendon in the front and center

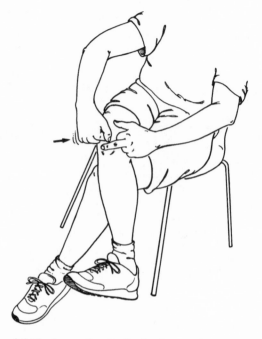

Figure 14. (A) The knee reflex: Strike the front and center of the leg one finger's width below the kneecap.

of the leg just below the kneecap (Figure 14A). The lower part of this leg should swing up. Repeat the test five to ten times. Then recross your legs so that the other knee is on top, and do the test all over again. Did each lower leg swing out about the same distance and with the same velocity? That's the expected, normal response. A reflex of normal strength on both sides suggests there is no neurological cause for your pain.

Ankle   Sit the same way in the same chair as for the knee reflex test. Cross your legs. Bend the knee of the leg on top, bringing the ankle toward yourself. Relax your foot so that it is loose and moves easily. Use your knuckles to strike your Achilles tendon in the center of the back of your ankle, just above the junction between your foot and calf (Figure 14B). Your foot should push down, so that it moves as

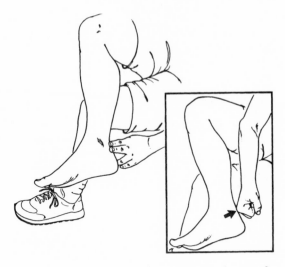

*Figure 14. (B) The ankle reflex: Tap the Achilles tendon two fingers'
width above the heel bone.*

though you were stepping on a car's gas pedal. Repeat taps five to ten
times. Recross your legs and test the other foot. Compare the results.

For both knee and ankle tests, if there's only a slight difference between the reflex on one side and the other, or you can't tell if there's
a difference, then you haven't discovered pathology. If there's a dramatic discrepancy—if tapping the knee, for example, makes that leg
fly up briskly while there is no motion at all in the other leg, or if one
leg moves twice as fast or far as the other, it's likely that you have a
neurological problem.

TREATING MUSCULOSKELETAL KNEE AND FOOT WEAKNESS

Muscles get stronger by getting tired. Do the following exercises at
night, when muscles are already slightly fatigued—this gives them a
"head start." It's not a good idea to tire out muscles at the beginning
of a busy day. It increases the likelihood that what you're doing the
exercises to avoid—a fall and painful consequences—will occur.

When exercising, pay attention to safety. To prevent falling, station yourself between two chairs and hold on with your hands. If the exercise involves moving forward, make sure you have supports you can reach easily.

1. Knee Weakness   Squat between the chairs, bending both knees. Straighten knees to regain your original position. Try the same exercise bending and straightening only the weaker knee. Do this ten times daily.

2. Weakness in Extending the Ankle (Your Foot Slaps or Drags during Walking)   Being careful not to lose your balance, tip yourself backwards onto your heels. Walk forward on your heels until the outside of the calf tires.

3. Weakness in Pointing Toes   Stand on tiptoes and balance for ten seconds. Do this several times a day. Advance to doing the exercise on one foot.

Well-Known Neurological Causes of Weakness

As with numbness and paresthesias, the pattern of weakness is a red flag for neurological difficulties. Reflexes are a good objective way of testing for nerve damage. The causes of this type of weakness have been worked out as they have for numbness and paresthesias. (See Figure 15 on page 152.)

There are differences, however, since the spinal cord and brain regulate many functions of peripheral nerves. The central nervous system houses nerve centers that keep reflexes at a healthy, controlled level. Therefore, after a stroke or spinal-cord injury there may be a paradox: the muscle is weak, but the reflex is abnormally strong. Here your commonsense determinations of "weak" and "strong" will lose their meanings, since you can have a strong reflex in a weak or even paralyzed muscle. These can occur after:

• Stroke—a cerebral hemorrhage or infarction (insufficient blood supply).

• Spinal-Cord Injury   Affects sensory nerves, motor nerves, or both. Spasm accompanied by paralysis can result from cutting off motor control from the restraining influence of higher control centers.

• Injury or Damage to Peripheral Nerves   Trauma, surgery and pressure produced by posture or position. This always reduces reflexes.

• Neuropathy   One or more nerves are damaged by systemic problems, reducing reflexes.

Numbness and paresthesias result from damage to sensory nerves that end on the skin. If the damage is at the root level, then numbness and paresthesias will be in specific areas called dermatomes. Motor nerve roots send impulses to particular sets of muscles called myotomes. The nerve-root symptoms chart (Figure 15 on page 152) shows the differences in these two types of areas and how they coordinate. Here are some examples of the patterns of nerve damage in the spinal cord producing weakness in the legs and feet:

• If the muscles at the back of the calf are weak or you have trouble walking on tiptoe on one or both sides, this could signal radiculopathy at L5-S1.

• If you can't walk on your heels or your foot drags or slaps the floor when you are walking, the L4-L5 nerve is probably involved.

• If your knee(s) buckle involuntarily or you have trouble rising from a sitting position, you should worry about L2 through L4.

• If walking tires your inner thigh, damage at L2 comes to mind.

Putting It All Together: Paresthesias, Numbness, and Weakness

Combining information about what you feel with what you can no longer do gives you overlapping clues about your diagnosis. When you analyze the knowledge you receive from your skin, your muscles, and your brain, the reward can be a useful understanding of the cause of your problem. In particular:

Weakness when it comes to pointing and walking on toes, and numbness on the outside of the calf and foot all signal difficulty at S1.

Weakness causing the foot to slap down during ordinary walking combined with pain, paresthesias, or numbness on the inside of the foot near the big toe and the inside of the calf suggests radiculopathy at L5.

When weakness, tingling, numbness and/or pain all occur at the knee, then L3 and L4 are a likely cause.

Weakness in bringing the legs together, and numbness and sensory changes in the upper inner thighs, point to an L2 nerve-root problem.

And sensory changes in the groin, combined with weakness in raising your leg (with the knee bent) and back pain at waist level should alert your doctor to a problem at L1.

I hope I have covered in the last three chapters the things that bother you most. If there is a pattern in your symptoms and/or signs that matches any of the descriptions I've given, then you have an idea about what could be wrong. The next question to answer is, Why?

CHAPTER 9

Major Causes of Chronic Low Back Pain

As mentioned in Chapter 5, musculoskeletal problems cause 85 percent of low back pain. Though these problems can be difficult to diagnose, and undiagnosed they may persist, the vast majority disappear spontaneously in three to four weeks. Now, for the 15 percent of patients who don't have musculoskeletal problems, and whose pain may become chronic, I'll describe the other, most common conditions and their symptoms and give some treatment advice.

Referred Pain

The concept of referred pain is basic to understanding neurogenic or neurological pain. (What people call pinched nerves, trapped nerves, and compressed nerves fall into the category of neurological pain.) This profoundly important fact about the way nerves work has a rather simple explanation.

All your life your brain has been receiving signals from your nerves. This has taught you to identify specific signals with particular locations. Obviously, if you're hammering a nail and your finger accidently gets in the way, you'll feel a big ouch in that finger. What's less obvious is that the same nerve can be stimulated anywhere along its course—in your shoulder, for example—and your brain will still locate the sensation in that finger.

This idea also applies to the lower back. The point of the injury may be in your spine, but you may feel the symptom in a distant location. For instance, if the sciatic nerve fibers that serve the bottom of the foot are injured, even if the injury is in the spinal canal, you will experience the pain, tingling, or numbness as coming from the bottom of the foot.

Two Kinds of Neurological Problems: Radiculopathy and Spinal Stenosis

Two neurological conditions that are often associated with low back pain are radiculopathy and spinal stenosis (see Figure 4, page 72). Both of these result from nerves being compressed as they pass through narrowed openings. Though they are different in nature, radiculopathy and spinal stenosis both affect nerves that travel down the leg and can produce sciatica (see Figure 7, page 97). Each of these problems has many underlying causes, which I'll discuss one by one below. A herniated disk, osteoarthritis, a trauma like a gunshot wound, a fracture, or a tumor—all of these can generate these two conditions.

Radiculopathies are reductions in the size of the small openings, called neuroforamina, through which nerve roots must pass as they exit the spinal canal. Spinal stenosis is a reduction of the inside diameter of the spinal canal itself.

SYMPTOMS AND SIGNS

If you have a radiculopathy or spinal stenosis, you usually have symptoms and signs along the path of the affected nerve fibers whose branches eventually connect to muscles and skin. For example, a radiculopathy of the nerve root at L5 may cause tingling between the first two toes and the outside top of the foot (Figure 15). In addition, it might lead to a gait disorder—the foot slapping rather than connecting smoothly with the ground during walking.

Spinal stenosis or radiculopathy can make one of your legs a little cooler or paler than the other. Your reflexes might be reduced. You might experience changes in bowel or bladder habits, with increased nighttime frequency of urination or leakage of urine when you cough or laugh.

DISTINGUISHING CHARACTERISTICS

These two conditions do, however, have differences. A radiculopathy occurs at a specific nerve root, but spinal stenosis can occur in a length of the spinal canal and may affect multiple rootlets. In other words, a single narrowing of the spinal canal at L3 is just one location of stenosis, but it can affect the nerve roots on the right at L5-S1 and on the left at L4.

If you have stenosis, you probably find your pain is more or less the same whether lying down or standing. Sitting might provide some relief.

٠ If you have a radiculopathy, the pain usually worsens when you sit, because sitting arches the back and raises pressure on the disk, compressing the nerve root as it exits the spine.

CAUTIONARY NOTE

The symptoms of stenosis or a radiculopathy occur in a pattern. Sometimes, however, what's compressed in a neurological situation

Nerve Root Symptoms Chart

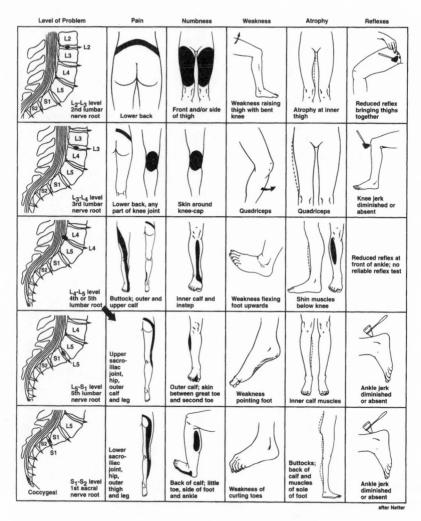

Level of Problem	Pain	Numbness	Weakness	Atrophy	Reflexes
L2, L3 L2-L3 level 2nd lumbar nerve root	Lower back	Front and/or side of thigh	Weakness raising thigh with bent knee	Atrophy at inner thigh	Reduced reflex bringing thighs together
L3, L4, S1 L3-L4 level 3rd lumbar nerve root	Lower back, any part of knee joint	Skin around knee-cap	Quadriceps	Quadriceps	Knee jerk diminished or absent
L4, L5, S1 L4-L5 level 4th or 5th lumbar root	Buttock; outer and upper calf	Inner calf and instep	Weakness flexing foot upwards	Shin muscles below knee	Reduced reflex at front of ankle; no reliable reflex test
L4, L5, S1 L5-S1 level 5th lumbar nerve root	Upper sacro-iliac joint, hip, outer calf and leg	Outer calf; skin between great toe and second toe	Weakness pointing foot	Inner calf muscles	Ankle jerk diminished or absent
L5, S1, S2, S1 Coccygeal S1-S2 level 1st sacral nerve root	Lower sacro-iliac joint, hip, outer thigh and leg	Back of calf; little toe, side of foot and ankle	Weakness of curling toes	Buttocks; back of calf and muscles of sole of foot	Ankle jerk diminished or absent

after Netter

Figure 15. Nerve-root symptoms chart: Since the Renaissance, the dissection of cadavers and surgical explorations of living people have enabled anatomists to chart nerve paths. This knowledge is fundamental to determining the exact location of radiculopathies, stenosis, and other nerve problems.

is neither nerves as they travel down inside the spinal canal nor roots that exit at various neuroforamina. Rather, it's the hard covering of the spinal cord, the dura mater. Pressure on the dura mater often results in patternless, helter-skelter symptoms in one or many locations, as well as burning, tingling, or other strange sensations.

WHAT TO DO

Steroidal and nonsteroidal antiinflammatory medications can reduce swelling and inflammation and therefore pain resulting from both radiculopathy and stenosis. However, before treating a painful condition, it's best to determine its cause.

Herniated Disk

WHAT IT IS

Herniated disk, slipped disk, or ruptured disk are familiar names for this common cause of serious low back pain, which studies say accounts for a little more than 11 percent of doctor visits for low back pain. The medical term for this condition is herniated nucleus pulposus (HNP).

No matter how it happens, a herniated disk always involves the breaking of an intervertebral disk so that some portion of it, or what was contained inside it, is pushed into space it wasn't meant to occupy. The presence of this hard or gelatinous disk material causes inflammation and swelling, often in the territory where nerves alone should be (Figure 16).

A herniated disk can create a radiculopathy or spinal stenosis, depending on whether the disk material blocks neuroforamina where nerve roots exit the spinal canal (a radiculopathy), or reduces space in the canal itself (spinal stenosis), affecting multiple nerve roots.

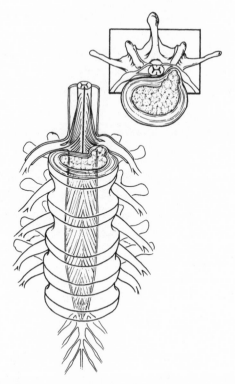

Figure 16. When a disk is herniated, some of its inner material escapes into regions usually reserved for nerves.

History

"When I moved my niece's refrigerator, something popped in my back," is the sort of report I typically hear from patients with a herniated disk. Several patients have come to me after herniating disks while reaching down and pulling one more weed from the garden.

Some things that cause herniated disks are lifting heavy objects, intense, unusual and/or violent twisting movements and an extended stay in a compromising position—for example a tall person bending forward for too long in a small car. Any activity or event that puts pressure or strain on the lumbar spine can be responsible, but often nothing specific can be identified.

Chances are your herniated disk will be most painful on one side in its early days. Sharp pains, either constant or intermittent, and often sciatica, characterize this problem. The pain is sometimes of a neurological type, and feels like electric shocks along the course of the sciatic nerve: in the buttock, the back of thigh, the back and outside of the calf, the heel, the space between the first and second toes, the outside of the top of the foot, or the sole of foot. A herniated disk can also produce stiffness and pain in the lower spine, or symptoms on the surface of the skin, including feelings of hot and cold, pinching, pins and needles, "bugs crawling," or other unusual sensations.

There may be alterations in what you feel—numbness, for instance, or hypersensitivity. Reflexes may also weaken or vanish. This type of neurological "insult" can cause the sympathetic nervous system to contract arterial blood vessels and make the affected limb cooler and paler than its mate.

The most common place for a herniated disk to occur is at L4-L5. When it does, it usually affects the L5-S1 root. This is a radiculopathy that results in symptoms on the skin of the outer calf, between the first and second toes, and possibly the last one or two toes. You may be weak when curling your toes and pointing your foot downward. Also, the Achilles tendon reflex in the affected leg will lose vigor. Sitting or lifting may intensify the pain.

If the disk herniates inside the vertebral canal, it can affect nerve fibers from one or more roots, possibly on both sides of the spine. This is spinal stenosis. It hurts more when standing than when sitting. Stenosis produces symptoms and signs in the patterns described in Figure 15. By looking at the chart you may identify one or more of the pattern of your symptoms and signs, which will suggest a diagnosis of radiculopathy or spinal stenosis or both.

Self-Examination

These simple procedures, which you can do at home, will indicate whether you have nerve damage that may be due to a herniated disk.

1. Test the weakness of muscles and reflexes of the affected side against the (often normal) other side by walking on tiptoes and heels. Weakness on tiptoe indicates a problem in the nerve roots at L5-S1; weakness walking on your heels, at L4-L5.

2. Gauge quadracep muscle strength by standing behind a chair and holding onto its back; deeply bend first one knee and then the other. If there is weakness, the difficulty can be traced to nerve roots at L2, L3, and L4.

3. Compare sensation region by region (for example, feet and then calves, and so forth) on the right and left by gently probing with a clean pin or other sharp object. If both sides are affected, you can compare your arms with your legs, the soles with your palms, the outsides of your upper arms with the outsides of your thighs, and so on.

4. In a lying-down position, straighten and raise the affected leg. With a herniated disk, pain will begin at least 20 degrees lower than with the other leg. Normally you should feel no pain below 80 degrees.[1]

5. Test for differences in your ankle reflexes by tapping on each Achilles tendon, which connects the calf muscles to the heel. The reflexes on the unaffected side will be more vigorous; in the same way, test and compare knee reflexes with the straight edge of a ruler applied just below the bone of the kneecap.

---

[1]A reminder: The straight leg raise is also painful if you are suffering from meningitis, hip arthritis (which will cause pain with a bent knee as well), or piriformis syndrome (see page 167).

WHAT IT'S NOT

Unlike a problem of muscular, postural, or peripheral origin, you can't reproduce the pain of a herniated disk by pressing on the tender spot. The joints aren't affected. Massage does no lasting good. Submerging yourself in a warm bath provides little or no relief. Herniated disks don't cause rashes or other systemic symptoms like fever, nausea, or vomiting. With extremely severe pain that causes a systemic upset, however, there may be some diarrhea.

CAUTIONARY NOTE

Exaggerated stories about herniated disks involve the themes of incapacitating, continuing pain and surgically inclined but incompetent physicians. Contrary to urban folklore, if you have a herniated disk the medical world likely has what you need for dramatic relief or a complete cure. But we're getting ahead of the story.

First, it's not true that all herniated disks are painful. Recent studies (for example, by Harvard researcher Maureen C. Jensen, in the *New England Journal of Medicine* for July 14, 1994) suggests that 30 percent of people who experience no back pain have significantly abnormal disks. Second, it is a myth that most slipped disks require surgery. Sometimes it is clear that the disk should be surgically removed. But 60 to 70 percent of herniated disks can and should be handled without using a scalpel. If pain continues unabated for six weeks, it's time for a surgical consultation. A decision in favor of surgery shouldn't cause undue anxiety. According to Augustus White and Manohar Panjabi, in their text *Clinical Biomechanics of the Spine,* depending on the suitability of the patient's problem, as many as 60 to 90 percent of these common operations are completely successful.

WHAT TO DO

Diagnosis   A physical exam is the best way to diagnose a herniated disk. There are also excellent technological means of detecting this problem. One is the MRI (magnetic resonance imaging) technique, which subjects tissues to high magnetic fields and actually tilts molecules of water and fat in the tissues, the way iron filings tilt when exposed to a magnet. Then it measures the change in the electric field. The MRI produces an image in more than one plane, distinguishing disk from nerves, bones, and muscles. The outline of the disk is clear, and any breaks are apparent.

The CT (computerized tomography) scan uses X rays to compile visual cross sections of the spinal cord and is excellent for picturing bones but is less informative about disks. This is because X rays go right through many soft tissues without delineating them. Nerves, for instance, can't be pictured with a CT scan. To counter this problem, many doctors when performing an MRI or CT scan inject a radiopaque dye (one that shows up well on photographic images) into spinal fluid to increase the definition of the nerves and the sheaths that cover them. This test, called a myelogram, silhouettes specific areas where disks, nerves, and bones come together. Dents in nerve tissue make the precise location of any neurological damage more visible. Regular X rays and a special type of "slice" X ray called a tomogram are also used to examine the spine.

The diagnostic tests I've just outlined give a detailed picture of what your back looks like inside. Let me stress again that you can have both pain and a herniated disk, and the two may be unrelated. These imaging techniques can tell you if you have a disk that's herniated, but they can't really determine whether it's the disk that your pain is coming from. Another test, called an EMG (electromyograph), measures nerve conduction and can record characteristic signals given off by muscles whose nerves are pinched or severed. An EMG can determine whether there really is nerve damage, can pinpoint its location, and therefore can scientifically connect a herniated disk with your actual pain.

After you see an orthopedist, a neurologist, or a physiatrist (a doctor of physical medicine and rehabilitation) to confirm a diagnosis of a herniated disk, you might try conservative measures.

Treatment   The first of these conservative measures is doing nothing, at least for a while. Take over-the-counter nonsteroidal antiinflammatory painkillers, and see what happens for three days to a week, depending on the severity of the pain. Dr. Douglas W. Wilmore, in an article titled "Catabolic Illness" (September 1991), has shown that remaining inactive for a week reduces muscle strength up to 20 percent, yet exercise programs improve strength no more than 10 percent per week. That means before one week of rest, the patient is three weeks away from normal. Some experts (see D. O. Porterfield and R. J. DeRosa's *Mechanical Low Back Pain*) cogently argue that while inactivity might not decrease low back pain, it will surely increase disability. I believe in the happy medium. Take it easy so as not to aggravate your pain, but don't weaken yourself by taking it too easy. A few days to a week at most.

For years the medical establishment laughed at another noninvasive way of dealing with herniated disks. This method, called the extension technique, is now widely accepted. In New Zealand, physical therapist Robin McKenzie stumbled on this way of relieving pain caused by a herniated disk more than ten years ago when he inadvertently kept a patient in a back-arched position for longer than usual. Since then he has developed and refined his system so that now he achieves a satisfactory result in 65 percent of his herniated disk cases. McKenzie's mechanical body techniques, which include stretching, "side gliding," physical positionings, and exercise, actually appear to return the displaced, irritating material of the slipped disk into its original, proper position: in line with the vertebral column and out of the way of the nerves.

Though herniated disk is a structural problem, another approach is musculopostural. Dr. John Sarnow of the Rusk Institute of Reha-

---

Dɪᴅ Yᴏᴜ Kɴᴏᴡ?

A survey of 293 physical therapists done by researchers at the University of Washington in Seattle concluded the majority believe Robin McKenzie's approach is the most useful for treating back pain.

Did You Know?

According to a major research study, 61 percent of HNP patients improved during the first year without surgery and 90 percent benefited from an operation. These patients were followed up four years later, when 86 percent who had not had surgery were better and 89 percent who had been operated on showed improvement. Amazingly, ten years later, no patients in either group had any symptoms of herniated disk!

---

bilitation and others have done fine work on stress reduction and its effect on posture, general body tone, and low back pain. Stress reduction through relaxation, imagery, breathing techniques, stretching, and other methods can have uncanny success, if not in eradicating the pain of a herniated disk, then in drastically reducing it.

When mild, noninvasive measures have failed and pain is severe and continuing, you may be a good candidate for more aggressive treatment. The thought of surgery makes most people nervous, but in reality it's one of the best-understood and most reliable remedies for severe back pain due to herniated disk. There are many precautions that can be taken before, during, and after surgery to assure its effectiveness, and I can highly recommend this form of treatment in many instances. I've been present at more than two hundred back surgeries and have seen only one minor and temporary abnormality that resulted from the operation.[2]

In spite of quite severe pain, some people are able to go about their daily lives and their normal activities. After a time, it could be as long as two years, many patients find that the pain just goes away. Often the herniated disk is still identifiable on the MRI, but the symptoms have

---

[2]The safety of surgery can be significantly enhanced if somatosensory evoked potentials (SSEPs) are done. Electrodes are attached to the patient's foot and head to monitor nerve function during the operation, helping surgeons avoid unnecessary injury to the spine.

---

disappeared. There are no reliable statistics on how frequently this happens, and obviously if your pain is severe, you should see a health-care professional. Pain that worsens when you are lying down also calls for medical attention, because it might indicate the presence of a tumor.

Spondylolisthesis

WHAT IT IS

This condition is the slippage of a vertebra forward and out of alignment relative to the vertebrae below it. Spondylolisthesis usually occurs in the forward-sloping lower lumbar vertebrae, and pain worsens during any movement that increases the misalignment. Physicians grade this according to the discrepancy in alignment: grade I is up to 25 percent, grade II is 25 to 50 percent, and so on.[3]

Spondylolisthesis can and often does simultaneously cause several problems. It can narrow the inside of the spinal canal (spinal stenosis) and/or the exits for nerves (radiculopathy). This usually occurs when the patient has a rating higher than grade I.

Almost invariably, spondylolisthesis is accompanied by spinal instability. Since the entire spinal column and the body above it is much less solidly supported, the instability prompts muscles to tighten painfully in response.

---

[3]Lateralisthesis is slippage to the side rather than forward; it has the same grading system.

HISTORY

Spondylolisthesis usually begins abruptly. A fall or other accident that breaks off the facet joints (where vertebrae connect to each other) allows that injured vertebra and all those above it to slip out of alignment. This slippage can also occur gradually, when joints become misshapen in cases of severe degenerative joint disease. Some believe spondylolisthesis can be a congenital defect.

SYMPTOMS AND SIGNS

An Olympic fencer came to me with this problem. She was suffering the type of neurological symptoms associated with spinal stenosis and radiculopathy, but the symptoms were relatively mild. More seriously, her muscles tightened painfully in response to movement. She experienced severe, intermittent, aching pain in her back and buttocks when she arched her back to protect her position during swordplay or lunged forward with her foil. I suspected spinal misalignment as the cause of her pain and that she had a classic case of spondylolisthesis. A simple X ray confirmed the diagnosis.

WHAT IT'S NOT

Spondylolisthesis is not a fracture or a spinal-cord injury. While it can cause neurological difficulties, it is usually a musculoskeletal problem with a musculoskeletal solution.

CAUTIONARY NOTE

The physical exam usually turns up nothing but muscles in spasm. Physicians may decide to treat the condition with nonsteroidal anti-inflammatory medication or trigger-point injections (both described in Chapter 11), assuming that, since there is no apparent cause the medication will help the problem go away by itself. Though this basically musculoskeletal condition can be at the bottom of some neurological problems leading to pain, when X rays show mild or moderate spondylolisthesis, doctors may conclude mistakenly that there is no neurological damage and therefore nothing can be done. But good evidence (from G. A. Schneiderman, writing in the journal Spine, August 15, 1995) supports the idea that there can be a local neurological source of pain in the back itself.

What to Do

The Olympic fencer used a brace called a lumbosacral corset, which relieved instability and neurological symptoms simultaneously. She worked at strengthening abdominal muscles and changed her thrusting technique slightly. These measures reduced her pain greatly, even during her most challenging competitions.

Physical therapy can do a lot for victims of spondylolisthesis. These patients work at improving posture, especially while walking; loosening tight muscles; and strengthening abdominal, flank, and back muscles so they can act as natural braces to prevent slippage and pain.

Surgery is sometimes an option to correct the alignment of vertebrae in an extreme case of spondylolisthesis, usually grade II or above.

Osteoarthritis[4]

What It Is

Osteoarthritis (degenerative joint disease) comes from normal and abnormal wear and tear on the joints and accounts for even more vis-

---

[4]When doctors refer to degenerative joint disease, they usually mean osteoarthritis. However, rheumatoid arthritis (see page 190) is also a degenerative process involving the joints.

its to the doctor than herniated disk does. Throughout our lives, most of our cells die and are replaced in a normal cycle. For example, beneath skin cells that we slough off regularly, there is a layer of tissue that is always making new skin. When cartilage-producing cells of the joints are injured by normal wear and tear, their secretions form slightly irregular surfaces in the joints. This starts a process that leads to further irregularity, deformation, pain, and damage (see Figure 17).

Degenerative joint disease consists of structural changes around the joint and does not affect nerves directly. Joints can develop abnormalities in the form of vertical growths called osteophytes, which resemble cave formations. In more serious cases of complicated os-

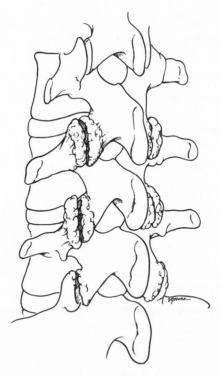

Figure 17. Joints deformed by osteoarthritis are often unstable and painful.

teoarthritis, neurological effects result from these structural changes in the bones that are sufficient to narrow the openings through which nerves must travel, both inside the spinal canal (spinal stenosis) and/or as they exit the spinal canal (radiculopathy).

HISTORY

This condition develops slowly, with aging, in everyone. Athletes and others who lead physically vigorous lives often fall victim to it earlier and with greater severity.

A circus strongman once came to me for morphine to ease the pain of his osteoarthritis. At age 45 he couldn't move his lower back at all without extreme sciatic pain. It hurt even more when he was performing. "The weight is nothing," he said. "It's the bending down I can't bear." I treated him with small success by trying to help him increase mobility in the joints above and below the area misshapen by the disease.

SYMPTOMS AND SIGNS

Sometimes osteoarthritis just causes joint pain in the spine that's worse in the morning. With simple osteoarthritis you get a constant ache or gnawing pain. If this condition becomes more serious, bony growth narrows neuroforamina and nerve roots get involved. The pain from nerve roots compressed as they exit neuroforamina in the spine is often shooting or stabbing. It follows the referred-pain pattern of radiculopathy I discussed earlier in this chapter. (See Figure 15 on page 152.)

Range of motion is reduced and is more painful at the limits of movement of the arms, the legs, and the spine, for example, when lifting. It's difficult to adjust your spine to maximize your strength.

WHAT IT'S NOT

Pain doesn't skip from side to side. It is rarely intermittent. No abrupt event causes the pain. Osteoarthritis is not a disease that strikes young people.

CAUTIONARY NOTE:

Some people use diuretics on the theory that a body with less fluid puts less pressure on inner structures and therefore experiences less pain. That's an extreme, potentially dangerous way of treating degenerative joint disease. Also I don't believe in steroid injections, which could further damage already vulnerable joints.

WHAT TO DO

Aspirin and nonsteroidal antiinflammatory medications can reduce swelling and pain, whether neurological, or, more commonly, arthritic. Combining simple remedies can be effective. Use a sequence of heat, gentle stretching exercises, and ice. Then analyze the movements that might increase pain so you can avoid them. If these means fail, there may be a neurological cause.

An EMG can help the physician distinguish between radiculopathy and spinal stenosis, which call for opposite treatments. Back arching and McKenzie exercises (see Chapter 11) are recommended for radiculopathy. Williams flexion exercises, which consist of forward bends and assuming the fetal position, often help reduce the pain of spinal stenosis. Administered by an especially skilled physical therapist or physician, degenerative joint disease may respond well to manual medicine techniques.

The strongman mentioned earlier would have none of these. Finally I succeeded in convincing him to make his act more dramatic by adding four assistants. These healthy young men brought out the barbells and lifted them to navel height, so my patient wouldn't have to bend and activate his pain. When I saw him last, he was off medication, performing with renewed zest.

Since arthritis is generally widespread and progressive, surgeons don't like to operate unless there's a particularly serious problem at a specific, identifiable point, such as a hip, which can be replaced. An MRI is necessary only if surgery is being considered.

Piriformis Syndrome

WHAT IT IS

This form of painful sciatica is caused by the piriformis muscle in one or both buttocks compressing the sciatic nerve.

Before 1934, piriformis syndrome was considered a major cause of sciatica. That year Drs. W. J. Mixter and J. S. Barr published an article in the *New England Journal of Medicine* showing that pain going down the leg could come from a problem in the spinal cord, where that nerve originates. The article was big news then, and it was the beginning of a powerful trend in medical thinking. Today many doctors believe *all* pain that goes down the leg must come from a cause in the spinal cord. I don't agree.

When I first discovered a simple test that confirms or rules out piriformis syndrome, some of my colleagues denied that anything but pathology in the spine could cause sciatica. In my opinion it stands to reason that at least some of the time (6 percent of the time, according to little-known studies done by Roger Hallin at the Mayo clinic about twenty years ago), pain going down the leg comes from something happening in the buttock. That "something," considering our anatomy, is usually the piriformis muscle compressing the sciatic nerve (Figure 18).

Unfortunately, people with this condition often spend years going from specialist to specialist without finding relief. Getting a diagnosis of piriformis syndrome can be difficult, because for so long it has been a diagnosis of exclusion. That is, doctors have had to rule

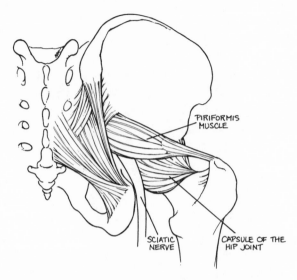

Figure 18. In piriformis syndrome the piriformis muscle compresses the sciatic nerve against underlying tissue.

everything else out and use deduction instead of objective tests to arrive at the diagnosis. Their attitude has been: "I've proved it's not anything else so it must be piriformis syndrome." That isn't true anymore.

In 1988, when I was working at the Albert Einstein College of Medicine, an orthopedic surgeon came to me with a patient, a hospital worker, whose pain he couldn't relieve. All tests were normal. He suspected piriformis syndrome, the obscure entity first written about two hundred years ago, and requested that I do an EMG. That, too, showed nothing. Frustrated, but suspecting my colleague's opinion about the case was correct, I put the patient in the FAIR test position, flexing, adducting, and internally rotating her thigh. This stretched the piriformis muscle, compressing the sciatic nerve between the muscle and the pelvic bone. The patient said, "That's it. That's the pain I feel." Then I did the H-Reflex test, a simple electrophysiological version of the Achilles tendon response. That first time I saw a greatly delayed reflex and felt sure I had discovered an objective diagnostic test for piriformis syndrome.

Not long afterward I saw a patient referred to me from a world-famous cancer center. This lovely woman had cancer invading her spinal cord and bowel. Doctors had implanted radium in her uterus to kill cancer cells. On top of all this she had a herniated disk. The pain was excruciating, and there were three really good possible explanations for her suffering. Unfortunately nothing had helped.

Thinking about her symptoms, I wondered if there could be a fourth, unidentified problem: piriformis syndrome. I decided to do the H reflex test. In ten minutes I knew that in addition to everything else, this woman had piriformis syndrome that could be treated. Physical therapy and home exercises brought my brave patient substantial relief until her death two years later.

History

People who sit in one position all day—stockbrokers; truck, bus, and car drivers; and computer programmers are prime candidates for piriformis syndrome. A patient of mine who fell asleep on the toilet seat after a Saturday night of drinking woke up Sunday morning with more than a hangover; he had also developed piriformis syndrome.

Sports like golf and tennis can cause this problem (right handers usually get it on the left side). A bad fall can be responsible. It can begin with aerobic exercise, come up from time to time, and then appear more frequently until the pain is constant. Poor gait, too much exercise, and leg-length discrepancy are also factors.

Symptoms and Signs

Pain along the course of the sciatic nerve characterizes this problem. The pain is usually worse when sitting than when standing. Piriformis syndrome is often particularly troublesome early in the morning, especially for those patients who sleep on their backs.

There is tenderness in the buttock. It can be difficult or can hurt to cross the painful leg over the other leg. Numbness, tingling, weakness, loss of reflexes, strange sensations, temperature discrepancies can develop in the parts of the body served by nerves from L4-L5, S1, especially when sitting (see Figure 15 on page 152). Often people have pain at a spot in the mid-groin, even producing tingling in the testicle or labia majora (the outer lips of the vagina). One in ten piriformis syndrome victims has pain on both sides.

Even when spondylolisthesis, sacroiliac joint derangement, or a radiculopathy are present, pain may be due to piriformis syndrome. It takes very little time and effort for the trained physician to find out by performing the diagnostic H-Reflex test.

What It's Not

Without a particular area of tenderness and pain in the mid-buttock, it's not piriformis syndrome. If you have a radiculopathy or spinal stenosis, you can feel a pain in your buttocks. This is not necessarily piriformis syndrome. However, if you have both a radiculopathy and piriformis syndrome, sometimes pain is relieved by curing piriformis syndrome. Try lying down, straightening the affected leg, and raising it 80 degrees off the bed or floor; if this action isn't painful, look for another cause.

Cautionary Note

I've found five tumors in patients suspected of having piriformis syndrome. These people (fewer than 1 percent of the patients I examined for this problem) had pain in the buttocks that went down the leg. The reason was not spasm in the piriformis muscle, but the tumor compressing the sciatic nerve. Some warning signs were weight loss and pain that was worse lying down rather than sitting.

What to Do

Piriformis syndrome responds well to conservative treatment. An injection of a small quantity of steroids and local anesthetic often relaxes the piriformis muscle, which reduces all pressure, and the pain often goes away almost magically. When this treatment has been successful, patients have cried with gratitude. Of course, that doesn't always happen. The shot will provide a complete cure only about 10 to 15 percent of the time. In my experience an injection gives 80 percent of patients relief for one to three weeks, during which time a program of physical therapy has time to take hold.

When the injection helps, physical therapy has an advantage: the relaxed muscle can be stretched more easily. Right after the shot the patient should begin physical therapy followed for as long as necessary by exercise at home for five minutes a day (see Chapter 11). Early results from small doses of injected botulinum toxin type A are encouraging.

Of the 723 cases of piriformis syndrome I've treated to date, 60 percent have improved by at least 60 percent within three months.

Sacroiliac Joint Derangement

What It Is

As far as I know, sacroiliac joint derangement is the most commonly underdiagnosed cause of low back pain. One reason is that this condition doesn't show up on X rays, MRIs, or EMGs.

We humans are prone to sacroiliac joint derangement because the entire spine and all its related structures rest on the spade-shaped sacrum, a midline bone which comes to a point where the coccyx begins. The sacrum is connected on both sides to the iliac bones, forming the right and left sacroiliac joints. The whole weight of the body above the waist is supported by those two joints.

In much of the animal kingdom, from the elephant to the mole, joints that must bear heavy weights are horizontal, like the top of a table. The knee and ankle are examples. But because we stand erect our sacroiliac joints are nearly vertical. In an engineering sense this isn't ideal. All the weight in the upper body, all our twists and moves, must be supported by these vertical joints, which routinely withstand tremendous forces but also can slip out of alignment rather easily.

By far the most likely cause of injury to our bones in general and our sacroiliac joints in particular is the stress we put on them with our activities. Our daily struggles with our environment that cause us to run, stop short, pull, push, lift, and so forth, put much more strain on us than gravity does.

The three-dimensional structure of the sacroiliac joint is very complex and irregular (Figure 19). Its normal range of motion is so small it must be measured in millimeters. You can think of the sacroiliac joint as a complicated three-dimensional jigsaw puzzle with numer-

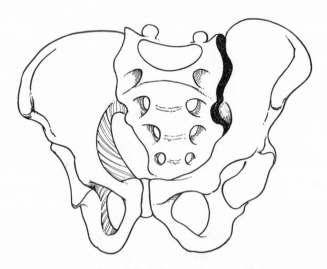

Figure 19. An inner view of the left sacroiliac joint. If the joint on one side of the sacrum is in poor alignment, the other side must be too.

ous notches and tabs that must fit exactly into one another. When the pieces don't match up perfectly, the result can be extremely painful.

Pushing any one part of this intricate structure beyond its normal range of motion might redistribute all the weight it bears, concentrating the weight on one tiny irregularity in the wall of the joint. That can be extremely painful until one changes position. If the angle or tilt of one side of the sacroiliac joint shifts, the patient may experience short bursts of pain on the other side. The pain usually occurs along the margins of the joint, but is sometimes so severe that it spreads to the hip or the abdomen or results in sciatica. Pressing on the joint usually hurts, at least to a degree. Sacroiliac joint derangement can cause all kinds of neck and back problems and frequently coexists with piriformis syndrome.

HISTORY

Think of recent events in your life that involved lugging heavy objects, posture-changing, emotional stress, or an accident involving feet or pelvis during exercise or dancing. A discrete, relatively minor, vertical trauma can cause sacroiliac joint derangement—for example, walking down the street and stepping in a pothole. Differing leg lengths can cause and also result from it.

SYMPTOMS AND SIGNS

Like spinal stenosis (and unlike radiculopathy), the pain from this condition can change from side to side. Characteristically the grinding or gnawing ache worsens with certain movements, such as lifting the feet when getting into or out of a car, reaching up while standing, bending down while knees are locked, and getting out of bed in the morning. Twisting to one side will hurt more than twisting to the other. This pain occurs below the iliac crests—just below the small

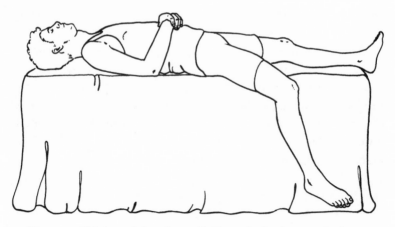

Figure 20.   If it hurts below the small of your back when your leg hangs off the bed, you have sacroiliac joint derangement. Carefully try the test on both sides.

of the back, where people used to talk about feeling lumbago. The pain occasionally can radiate down the leg, like sciatica, but lacks the objective signs of nerve involvement. Shifting your weight usually helps a little but doesn't alleviate the pain for long.

Look for pain that can get worse all of a sudden at any time of the day. One leg might feel shorter than the other. You can find it difficult to spread your legs apart.

Self-Examination   If lying down on your back with one leg hanging off the bed causes pain in this joint, you are probably suffering from SI derangement (Figure 20).

What It's Not

With sacroiliac joint derangement, there aren't any neurological signs: no numbness, weakness, or change in reflexes. A patient rarely experiences sensations of hot and cold, or tingling. If the pain hasn't been bad all day, it's unlikely that it will wake you in the night.

Cautionary Note

The pain of sacroiliac joint derangement is always in the lower back, but some patients mistakenly think it's in their hips. Failure to look for this problem is a usual cause of the failure to diagnose it. If the derangement is relatively new, it can be cured quickly.

What to Do

Unfortunately, standard diagnostic tests don't show sacroiliac joint derangement, but they can be helpful in ruling out other problems. An MRI of the lumbar and sacral regions of the spine can rule out a fracture, herniated disk, and spinal stenosis. EMGs, bone scans, myelograms, and gallium scans (see Chapter 11) are usually of little use. Abscesses due to tuberculosis and other infectious diseases can reach the sacroiliac region and mimic derangement.

What you need is a physician who can recognize this problem through a complete set of hands-on tests. In one of these relatively simple tests the physician places his or her thumbs on the patient's pelvic bones just above and beside the sacrum. When the patient bends forward, in standing and sitting positions, the doctor can feel the derangement.

I recommend an osteopath who is willing to work with you by using actual physical manipulation. Physiatrists and physical therapists are next on my list as sources of help. Strain/counterstrain techniques used in manual medicine, muscle energy techniques, and methods of intentional muscle fatigue can bypass the usual fixed rigidity caused by bone displacement and open up the possibility of manipulation, which can put the joint in its proper place.

Surgery is done, but only in cases of severe derangement or severe fracture.

Fracture

WHAT IT IS

A bone break, though it might only be a tiny corner of the bone or a crack in the bone, can be terribly painful. This is because the periosteum, the thin transparent bone covering, is richly invested with nerves.

HISTORY

A break in a spinal vertebra usually occurs in one of two ways:

1. Severe trauma like a bad fall from a horse or an automobile accident can, of course, cause a fracture.

2. In older people, particularly if osteoporosis is present, fractures in vertebral bodies can occur with mild repetitive strain or appear spontaneously.

SYMPTOMS AND SIGNS

In either type of fracture there may or may not be neurological signs, depending on where the break occurs. Classic symptoms of spinal fractures with neurological involvement are numbness of toes and weakness or the inability to move part or all of one or both legs or feet. Fractures in the lower spine reduce or abolish reflexes. A fracture above T_{11}-T_{12} heightens reflexes and spasm. With spontaneous or other fracture of the vertebral body, pain that is already terrific worsens when you bend forward, and may be relieved by lying down.

Usually when a fracture occurs in a vertebral body, the pain is due to the pressure of muscle pull and gravity. Therefore, arching the back and taking the weight off the vertebrae relieves pain.

WHAT IT'S NOT

You feel no pain, numbness, or weakness above the level of the fracture. Arching rarely increases pain. The fracture causes no pain when pressure is applied to muscles only. Lying down hardly ever makes a fracture hurt more.

CAUTIONARY NOTE

If you think you or someone you encounter has an acutely broken back, movement could cause further damage. While the injured person's head is supported, he or she should roll, or be "log-rolled," onto a door or stretcher, be secured so there is no movement, and be taken to a hospital.

WHAT TO DO

If you have the history described above, you should get an X ray, which can diagnose fracture. After two or three weeks a process called demineralization makes very small fractures more visible on X rays.

There's always a big question with fractures: are they stable or unstable? Unstable fractures cause potentially dangerous misalignment of the spine, allowing for unnatural movement of the spinal column. This instability risks ripping nerves and causing other serious problems, and therefore requires quick medical intervention in the form of a cast or surgery.

If a fracture in a young person is stable, it will probably heal substantially in six to eight weeks if motion is sufficiently restricted. In older people with spontaneous vertebral body fractures a hyperextension brace will relieve pain and promote healing by keeping weight off the affected region. These small common fractures are usually stable.

Sometimes the most serious consequence of trauma isn't a fracture but swelling inside the spinal canal. If your X rays are normal after an automobile accident or any severe blow to the spine, but then you develop numbness, tingling, or any other neurological signs, see a doctor quickly.

Coccygodynia

What It Is

The coccyx, the five fused bones below the sacrum, can be broken or injured in a bad fall. As with a finger these bones connect to our bodies only at one end. Because of this, when one or more of these bones is broken or dislocated by direct trauma, movement isn't affected.

History

A backward fall that lands you on your buttocks can break your coccyx, as can an automobile accident or other traumatic event.

Symptoms and Signs

The pain, usually stabbing, can be severe. Sitting is usually a problem, because there is direct pressure right at the site of the fracture. However, there is seldom swelling with coccygodynia.

WHAT IT'S NOT

If there are any neurological signs or symptoms, they're not due to this condition. There may be pain with bowel movements, but there are no changes of bowel or bladder habits. Genital sex isn't affected. Because of its location and sensitivity, you may think you have hemorrhoids, but there's no blood.

CAUTIONARY NOTE

Women of childbearing age should have an X ray to diagnose this condition at about the time of the menstrual period so as not to endanger a fetus.

WHAT TO DO

A normal, inexpensive X ray is the best way to find out if coccygodynia is your problem. Sometimes the X ray will be negative, because the problem is not a break or crack in the bones but only a bruise of the periosteum.

Injection of a small amount of steroid just above the anus and right next to the affected bones can eradicate pain seven times out of ten. This kind of injection, usually done by a physiatrist, may last for only three months before something re-creates the pain. If that happens, another injection can be given.

Bursitis

WHAT IT IS

Bursas, like joint capsules, are pouches containing lubricant. Their function is to separate and protect muscles from one another or from bones. Bursitis occurs when a bursa becomes irritated and swells because of inflammation due to pressure or friction. Swollen bursas (Figure 21) cause a vicious cycle by getting in the way of the very tissues they're meant to separate, which increases the friction, swelling, and pain.

There are three relevant types of bursitis, which are named by location:

1. Ischial: bursas beside the bones on which you sit.
2. Trochanteric: bursas close to the bone of the hip.
3. Obturator internis: bursas associated with the muscle in the buttock behind and slightly above the ischial bones.

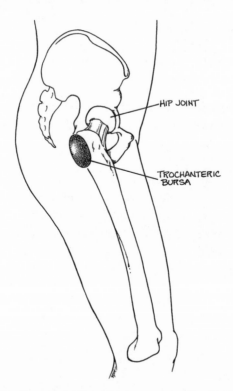

Figure 21. Trochanteric bursitis: Tenderness is confined to the area where the hip bone is nearest the skin.

History

Though it isn't always the case, bursitis can also result from trauma. Usually extra stress precedes the pain. For example, persistent sitting, lying, or sleeping on one side can set you up for trouble. Sometimes there are no historical clues. You have no idea what caused the pain or exactly when it began.

Symptoms and Signs

This condition isn't painful except when there is pressure on the affected region, and then the pain can be extreme. There are no objective signs apart from swelling, which is occasionally so exaggerated it can be detected by an X ray.

What It's Not

Bursitis is not a neurological disorder. There is no weakness, no numbness, no reduction in reflexes, and no strange sensations (paresthesias). If there is hip pain that goes inward to the groin, then the problem is in the joint, not the bursa.

Cautionary Note

The injections I recommend below can take a few days to work. If the steroid is mistakenly injected into the neighboring tendon, there could be serious and lasting damage.

What to Do

The answer to bursitis is an injection of steroid mixed with an anesthetic like lidocaine. In my experience this takes care of the problem with dramatic speed in as many as 90 percent of patients. Complications are very rare.

Swelling, Scarring, and Gynecological Problems

WHAT THEY ARE

Swelling increases the contents of any tissue in a given space. This limits the available room for the structures that normally occupy that space, putting pressure on them and crowding them, sometimes to the point of injury. While this is particularly true in the spinal canal, it also applies to the pelvis.

In the spinal cord, scarring or adhesions can be devastating. The presence of these tissues can choke off the blood supply to the nerve cells, causing muscle weakness, low back pain, and/or sciatica that is difficult to cure.

Scarring after a trauma or surgery also reduces space, but in the particular way in which tight, relatively intransigent bands of scar tissue can restrict the movement of other structures. Scarring can cause adhesions, which are bridges between two structures that are not normally connected, like two muscles or a muscle and skin.

HISTORY

A variety of conditions, including premenstrual syndrome (PMS), endometriosis (migration of tissue from the lining of the uterus to organs outside the womb), and pelvic inflammatory diseases (such as gonorrhea) can cause swelling. Pelvic congestion syndrome, a circulatory problem that occurs more commonly in women but might also have a male form, also results in swelling and consequent compression.

Scarring is usually the result of a particular event, often surgery. Pelvic inflammatory disease can also be responsible for scarring.

Symptoms and Signs

Low back pain is associated with all these problems. Swelling and scarring can cause irritation to nerves and classic neurological symptoms.

Fluid retention, particularly associated with PMS, can cause weight gain in the week before the menstrual period. Sometimes this kind of swelling is visible to the naked eye.

Internal scarring is difficult to pinpoint, since these bands of connective tissue can form in any location.

Lying down and raising your legs and pelvis as high as possible should temporarily relieve pelvic congestion syndrome.

What It's Not

These problems don't involve a fracture. They never show up on X rays. PMS and endometriosis have no neurological symptoms, and discomfort disappears with the onset of the menstrual period.

Cautionary Note

Tell your physician about any surgery you've undergone. Report on pregnancies. If pain is worse when lying down, possibly a tumor is involved.

What to Do

If you suspect a "female" problem, a gynecologist should look at you. However, to deal with low back pain your gynecologist might need consultation with a team that includes a surgeon and a physiatrist.

Exercise and reduction of salt intake are recommended for PMS and endometriosis. Meditation and other relaxation techniques can also provide relief. Prescription medications like Lupron and Ergot derivatives are used for these conditions and for pelvic congestion syndrome. Myofascial release and deep manual therapeutic techniques (see Chapter 3) have helped many patients. Doctors try to avoid surgery, since it can cause further scarring and new adhesions.

Facet Syndrome

What It Is

This topic is surrounded by controversy, but some believe facet syndrome results from inflammation of the facet joints in the spine and accounts for a great deal of low back pain. (See Chapter 1, p. 34, for a description of facets.)

History

Pain increases when you twist and bend simultaneously, and when arching backward after bending forward. Often the pain is localized in a given place. In many studies people with facet syndrome are middle aged or older and have a history of low back pain.

Symptoms and Signs

Pain can occur with pressure at a specific point. It often hurts more turning to one side than the other. An ordinary X ray can show a joint that is different from the others; sometimes a joint has swollen so much it resembles a mulberry. But X rays sometimes show joint abnormalities in patients who experience no pain, and sometimes patients who are experiencing pain have normal X rays.

What It's Not

Facet syndrome is mostly aggravated by changes in position. It usually doesn't affect the person when he or she is sitting, standing, walking, or lying down. There is no leg pain, not much pain with coughing or sneezing, and muscle spasm occurs only in the immediate area. There are no paresthesias and no numbness.

Cautionary Note

Some tumors of the joint can produce similar symptoms, but an X ray can pick them up.

What to Do

A diagnostic test can be the best treatment for this hard-to-diagnose condition. If an anesthetic like lidocaine is injected into the painful joint, it can relieve spasm and other conditions as well. The diagnosis can be made by injecting two anaesthetics that have two different durations. Monitoring the medicines and the time the patient experiences pain to arrive at a diagnosis has been championed by some physicians. Manual medicine in conjunction with injection and intermittent traction seem to work best.

Claudication

What It Is

This vascular disease strikes 3 million Americans, most of them over fifty years old. Claudication consists of pain in the backs of calves when walking and is the result of active muscles not getting adequate oxygen, food, and waste removal from circulating blood.

History: Symptoms and Signs

Walking a short distance produces pain in the backs of the calves. The pain disappears after a few seconds of rest and reappears again when walking the same distance.

What It's Not

Intermittent claudication isn't back pain, though it mimics spinal stenosis, which is also known as pseudo-claudication. This condition isn't sciatica; it does not involve nerves.

Cautionary Note

This generalized problem of arterial circulation often appears in legs when it's already quite advanced in the heart and brain.

What to Do

Develop a program that requires progressively more walking every day. This is effective in increasing mobility over a six-month period, directly adding to walking range, and in decreasing pain.

Herpes Simplex

What It Is

Herpes is a viral infection that is usually but not always sexually transmitted. It is believed that viral particles lodged in sensory nerve cells near the spinal cord migrate down specific nerves to their endings in the skin. This causes quite intense feelings of tingling, skin hypersensitivity to touch, severe pain, and outbreaks of small fluid-filled sores.

History

Herpes outbreaks are usually associated with emotional or extreme physical stress, which also can exacerbate musculoskeletal and other types of low back pain.

Symptoms and Signs

Sores called vesicles appear during the contagious stage, mature, and disappear together. The area of the symptoms can be similar to those of radiculopathy because they are in the distribution of a given nerve root. The pain, however is of a very different character. There's smarting or burning of the skin and tingling. Hypersensitivity can lead to pain even when clothing brushes against the affected limb.

What It's Not

This condition doesn't cause weakness or numbness, though herpes pain can make the victim reluctant to move. The pain it causes has nothing to do with position, except when position causes additional pressure on the skin.

Cautionary Note

Herpes symptoms can come and go for months or even years.

A few medicines, like acyclovir, can reduce the incidence and severity of herpes symptoms. In cases of extreme pain, transcutaneous electrical nerve stimulation (TENS) can provide relief of pain, which in turn lessens stress, often a primary cause of an outbreak of herpes.

Other Neurological Diseases: Neuropathy, Amyotropic Lateral Sclerosis, and Multiple Sclerosis

WHAT THEY ARE

These three generalized neurological conditions are not, strictly speaking, within the diagnostic territory of low back pain. They can, however, cause severe back pain.

Neuropathy   Just as eczema can affect part or all of your skin, a neuropathy can affect some or all of your nerves. When their sheaths are damaged, nerves conduct impulses poorly, dangerously altering sensation and coordination. When the nerve cells themselves are affected, the nerve fibers don't conduct at all, and sensation and strength are reduced.

Amyotropic Lateral Sclerosis (ALS)   This condition, also named for the baseball player Lou Gehrig, who made it famous, is like a sort of slow polio; it progressively affects and kills motor nerves but doesn't affect sensation or mental capacities. People with ALS generally have a life span after diagnosis of five to seven years. Low back pain results from muscle weakness of the lower extremities, abdomen, and back, and extreme constipation.

Multiple Sclerosis (MS)   Small protein deposits arise in nerves in the brain and spinal cord and interfere with nerve conduction. This disrupts basic nervous system function, including sensation, movement, coordination, balance, bowel and bladder performance, thinking, and often eyesight. Low back pain comes from sensory changes, clumsy movements and (like ALS) sitting in a wheelchair too long.

History

Neuropathy   This condition could be related to diabetes, renal or thyroid disease, or exposure to toxic substances or radiation.

ALS   The cause of this progressive disease is unknown, but it could be viral.

MS   An immune system abnormality is suspected of producing this disease. This disease has an erratic course, with symptoms increasing and decreasing in different limbs.

Symptoms and Signs

Neuropathy   Sensation and / or muscles weaken first in the feet and toes. Back pain may appear. Clumsiness may develop as a result of reduced sensation, reflexes, and motor control.

ALS   This disease comes on insidiously, with weakness and occasional tingling. Sensation isn't affected. Hand or foot muscles may twitch involuntarily (or in medical terminology, "fasciculate"). This usually starts in hands and forearms. Weakness progresses.

MS   Symptoms and signs show up in two or three limbs. A combination of sensory and motor symptoms include, for example, tingling in one leg and numbness in one arm, trouble controlling bowel and bladder, dimming vision in one eye, possible weakness in one leg, and loss of coordination.

WHAT IT'S NOT

Neuropathy   This condition is never caused by trauma; joint pain is very rare.

ALS   There is no numbness or change in sensation or pain. Usually mental processes are not affected.

MS   This disease is rare in people raised in warm climates.

CAUTIONARY NOTES

Neuropathy   This condition frequently has a treatable cause, but sometimes a cause cannot be found.

ALS   Occasional muscle twitches don't mean you have this disease.

MS   Today this disease can be detected in very mild forms; in these cases symptoms don't progress, and MS has no effect on the person's life.

WHAT TO DO

These are serious conditions, and if having read the descriptions of symptoms above, you suspect you have one of them, see a neurologist.

Rheumatoid Arthritis

WHAT IT IS

Many researchers think this condition is an autoimmune disease in which the body attacks the collagen in its own joint linings.

History

Rheumatoid arthritis can develop at any time in a person's life. Untreated or insufficiently treated streptococcal infections, such as strep throat or scarlet fever, are known causes. Nightshade vegetables—tomatoes and eggplant—make it worse. Joints often become visibly deformed over time.

Symptoms and Signs

Joints of fingers just above your knuckles are usually involved, as are joints in wrists, neck, ankles, and feet. Pain (accompanied by warmth in the joints) can come and go. Joint stiffness is a prominent feature.

What It's Not

Pain isn't due to neurological problems but to an autoimmune process. Adaptations to rheumatoid pain can cause musculoskeletal problems, which should be treated in addition to the underlying problem.

Cautionary Note

Blood tests that show the presence of rheumatoid factor (RF) and antinuclear antibody (ANA) are nearly diagnostic for rheumatoid arthritis; however, negative test results don't rule it out. Physical therapy can be damaging if the therapist doesn't know you have this condition.

What to Do

The first treatments for rheumatoid arthritis are physical and occupational therapy. They increase range of motion and reduce pain. If the disease progresses, steroids, gold, and chemotherapy are treatments of choice. Research on a new generation of drugs promises relief from this serious degenerative joint disease. Gentle physical therapy, environmental adjustments, and adaptive devices like elastic shoelaces that don't need to be tied or untied can make you more comfortable and more able to function.

Scoliosis

This condition, also called curvature of the spine, doesn't cause back pain. Medical intervention isn't necessary unless the curvature exceeds 20 degrees.

CHAPTER 10

Twenty-Four Tricks to Ease Your Aching Back

P ain and accompanying disability have unpleasant emotional consequences. Even the patients most determined to find relief sometimes give in to feelings of helplessness, frustration, and depression. In fact, there is hope for the majority of backache victims. I have been studying back pain for more than ten years, and I can say with certainty that the preponderance of my patients get substantial relief. Even more could change their depressed moods by seizing the opportunity to do what they can for themselves, without costly, formal medical attention. The most practical attitude is to gather information and then use it to gain as much control as possible over an unpleasant or disabling condition.

Recently I followed up on seven hundred patients who had come to me with back problems, including sciatica. On the average these people had suffered from pain for over six years. They had already seen an average of seven different practitioners in their search for a cure. All this had not been futile. This large patient group reported, on average, an improvement of 67 percent.

As mentioned earlier, a great number of patients get better by themselves, not because of any doctor's intervention. But most of the patients I saw hadn't improved sufficiently, even after the attentions of half a dozen doctors. For some, relief required proper diagnosis and treatment or courses of physical therapy, and a few had successful surgery. A large number of these patients, however, learned to manage their back problems themselves, with simple, inexpensive or cost-free techniques they used at home.

Experience has taught me that the twenty-four "tricks" that follow can provide, if not a permanent cure, then islands of painlessness that seem miraculous. These remedies are like basic first aid for your back, and you can experiment with one or all of them, shifting when necessary. You can also invent your own. In the process, you are bound to learn more about your physical condition, to ease your pain at least for the moment, and at the same time to fight the feelings of depression that so often accompany physical problems.

First, here are four super- or metatricks that can help every single person with back pain, regardless of its severity, duration, or type:

• Use Common Sense   I've had back pain myself, and been in such distress that at first I didn't think of the obvious. It took my wife to tell me to take aspirin.

• Know Your Problem   If you know what's wrong, you have a great advantage when devising and using home remedies.

• Don't Push Yourself Too Hard   Discontinue doing anything that makes your back hurt more or increases your symptoms.

• Don't Feel Guilty   "It's because of something dumb I did," is a common notion among people who suffer from back pain. The embarrassment keeps some from seeking help.

All the strategies that follow fit within the context of those four principles.

1. Use Over-the-Counter Painkillers

The value of taking over-the-counter medications like aspirin, ibuprofen, and other nonsteroidal antiinflammatories is grossly underestimated. I have found that for one reason or another patients who could benefit from these medicines simply don't use them. Some of these medications provide more than just symptomatic relief; they actually work to eliminate the cause of the pain. For example, two extra-strength (500 milligram) Ecotrin taken with food four times a day are not likely to cause stomach upset, but they will in many cases decrease inflammation and swelling caused by overactivity.

If you suspect your pain is caused by osteoarthritis, a musculoskeletal problem, or a sprain that might eventually heal on its own, it is certainly worth trying over-the-counter painkillers.

These nonprescription medicines are also effective when used in advance. For example, if you always have back pain the morning after playing tennis, take an antiinflammatory painkiller 24 to 36 hours before you arrive at the courts. This allows the medication to achieve a beneficial level in your blood before you start hitting the ball.

Take these over-the-counter products like their prescription counterparts—with meals—to avoid adverse effects on your stomach. These remedies aren't suitable for long-term daily use with chronic conditions, because they can cause ulcers. Overdose or prolonged use can damage kidneys.

Tylenol (acetominophen) isn't an antiinflammatory. This nonprescription painkiller reduces symptoms by acting on the central nervous system. Its efficacy is well documented, but the mechanism of its action isn't well understood. Tylenol isn't hard on the stomach, but unlike antiinflammatory medications it has no beneficial effect on the causes of pain in the back, muscles, and nerves. Too much or habitual use of this product is likely to harm the liver.

2. Lean Correctly

Ted, my upstairs neighbor, a lawyer and self-described workaholic, unexpectedly rang my doorbell one evening. "I came home from work early to lie down and rest my aching back," he told me. "But I'm in such bad shape I can't bend over to take off my shoes."

A short, informal physical examination turned up what I was quite certain was a combination of sacroiliac joint derangement and muscle strain, probably brought on by years of carrying a briefcase that weighed at least thirty pounds.

Half an hour later Ted became an expert in the technique of leaning. This simple exercise stretches the muscles between the pelvis and thoracic spine and works best when done for very short periods of time so it doesn't cause muscles to contract.

With a little instruction from me, Ted used his arms to support himself as he leaned forward against a tabletop until his stomach and back muscles relaxed enough to let gravity do its part. It took no more than a couple of minutes before he felt a definite click. I knew and he immediately understood that this was a signal. The leaning had realigned his sacroiliac joint and corrected the derangement. Though he still had to deal with muscle strain, Ted's sacroiliac pain had vanished.

How to Lean

Stand so close you are almost touching a kitchen counter, desk, table, or object of comparable height (Figure 22). Feet should be comfortably apart. With palms facing away from your body, lean forward slightly until your hands come to rest against the edge of the counter. As you lean forward, dig your elbows into your midsection so that your forearms support much but not all of your weight. Your legs

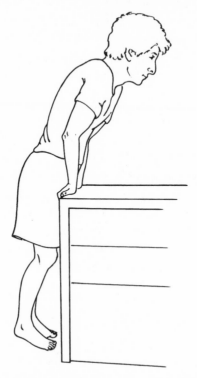

Figure 22. Leaning is often a miraculous cure for sacroiliac joint derangement.

should feel some relief from weight bearing as your heels lift slightly off the floor. Relax your abdomen. You're doing this exercise correctly if you feel a stretch in your lower back.

Lean for 5 to 20 seconds, as many times a day as you like. Rest either briefly or for long periods, whichever is more comfortable, before leaning again. This exercise can be done as frequently and for as long as you like. It takes practice to learn to do it properly.

Use leaning to relieve pain from sacroiliac joint derangement, a herniated disk, and musculoskeletal ailments. Leaning will not ease the pain of myopathy (generalized muscle disease) or spinal stenosis.

3. Curl Up in a Fetal Position

Curling up in the fetal position is good for the pain of a herniated disk, and for arthritis of the spine, muscle spasm, and premenstrual syndrome (PMS). Lie on your side in bed, and draw your knees up toward your chest. Put a pillow between your legs to reduce hip pressure and the pull of the legs on one side of your spine. Stay in this position as long as you want.

Pain can increase if you get too fierce and curl up too tightly or if your bed is so hard that it elevates your hips. Assuming this position can make the pain of a vertebral fracture worse; it can also aggravate tenderness in ligaments of the spinal cord.

4. Lose Weight

When his father had a heart attack and faltered, Paul, an architect, caught the older man in his arms, wrenching his back. The heart attack proved fatal for his father. Years later Paul's back still hurt so much some days that he couldn't get out of bed. He had a combination of problems: grief, the emotional symbolism of his pain's origin, an emotionally taxing job, and he was overweight.

I insisted my high-strung patient diet to lose 10 pounds and swim for exercise every morning before going to work. The weight loss reduced the load on his spine, and regular exercise strengthened his abdominal and spinal muscles so he didn't have to strain as much to keep his body erect. The whole routine helped Paul deal with emotional stress. The pain, while not completely vanquished, is now under good control.

HOW TO DIET

The best method I know for losing weight is the simplest. You can eat whatever you want and, within reason, whenever you want. The only restriction is that you must push your chair away from the table when you're still a bit hungry. Let's say you eat 5 to 10 percent less than you would to be utterly and totally satisfied.

This reduces your caloric intake. Even more important, as you eat less over a period of time, the smooth involuntary muscles of your stomach shrink slightly. Your smaller stomach feels sated with a smaller amount of food. Make a rule of ending a meal when you're 90 to 95 percent satisfied, and weight loss will continue until you reach your goal. You feel lighter and your level of mental and physical activity rises. When you have lost weight and your stomach is smaller, you should have little difficulty keeping pounds off.

A psychotherapist patient of mine from Atlanta had a double problem. She was overweight but her occupation kept her quite sedentary. Furthermore, her feet hurt so much she couldn't exercise in convenient ways. This woman lost 40 pounds in six months using the push-yourself-away-from-the-table technique; her smaller stomach and consequently diminished appetite has helped her keep the weight off. As a fringe benefit, her feet, previously swollen and almost too overburdened to support her firmly, have returned to normal.

5. Wear Proper Shoes

Shoes are some of the usual suspects in cases of back pain. Not only are shoes our foundation, we also use them as levers and cushions when we walk. Ill-fitting shoes influence our posture, just as foot abnormalities do, and often bring about backache. You should look at your shoes carefully, keeping in mind that a different pair or just another pair of shoes might cure the ache in your spine.

It's sad but true that some of the shoes considered most beautiful can hurt us most. High-heeled shoes bring weight forward, arching backs and causing pain, particularly in cases of spondylolisthesis. Narrow toes keep the body weight back, hurting people with sacroiliac joint derangement. You may say, "Good. I'll get high-heeled shoes with narrow toes, and everything will come out all right." Unfortunately, the combination will almost certainly create painful contortions and antics when you stand and walk. Look for comfortable footwear with good support.

Both high-heeled women's shoes and cowboy boots for all genders should fit well. But there is a related factor that *is* different for men and women. Researchers videotaping adults balancing on unstable surfaces found few differences between young and old, thin and fat, short and tall people. However, the sexes separated out neatly. Men maintained equilibrium by bending their knees and swinging their hips. Women balanced by tilting their ankles and repositioning their feet.

Each different gender style has the potential for backache. When men's hamstring muscles (the muscles in the back of the thigh) are tight, their hips can't function properly. This requires men to use their heads and torsos to balance, causing back pain. To the extent that women's shoes restrict their ankle range of motion, their buttock and trunk muscles must stiffen, a situation that could also result in backache.

People with diabetes and mild spinal-cord injury or pinched nerves in their backs sometimes have reduced feeling in their feet. They should be particularly attentive to possible problems with feet or shoes.

Podiatrists don't see patients for back pain, but by refitting shoes and caring for the ills of the feet they frequently help cure it.

6. Use Shoe Orthotics

Shoe orthotics are additions to footwear, inside or outside. They're designed to improve foot support, the way the foot bears weight and moves during walking. Orthotics can accommodate neurological dysfunctions, fractures, strains and sprains, and many kinds of foot abnormalities. They're valuable for gait and posture disorders, which are common causes of back pain. Physiatrists, orthopedists, and podiatrists can prescribe these inserts and shoe adjustments. Licensed orthotists can make them, but if you understand your problem, you might be able to find a premade orthotic that works for you at a pharmacy for half the price.

I've seen patients smile with disbelief (and relief) when a little shoe lift used for leg-length discrepancy instantly erased pain that had been there for years. Incidentally, if you have leg-length discrepancy (see Chapter 2 for the self-exam), you can try two, or even four, Dr. Scholl's insoles in your shoe. Turn over a left insole to fit it into the right shoe and vice versa.

7. Lift Correctly

There are two common mistakes in lifting. The first is using the wrong muscles—the back muscles. The powerful muscles of the buttocks and thighs are made for use when people are lifting heavy weights.

Ungraceful though it might appear, bend your knees when lifting heavy objects so that you have a solid foundation for your spine (Figure 23). Keep your trunk vertical. When your trunk is horizontal, the pressure against the lower back amounts to many hundreds of extra pounds. Even if the added force doesn't sprain or strain back muscles, it can compromise an intervertebral disk. The arms and bent waist form an unnecessarily long lever, and the disk becomes the fulcrum, a tiny section of which must bear the amplified, concentrated weight.

The second usual error is lifting an object far away from oneself. To lift an object without hurting your back, get close to it. When you're at a distance, the stress on your spine rises exponentially. This

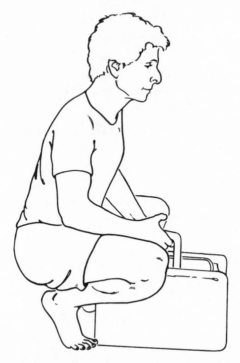

Figure 23. When lifting an object, keep it close to you and keep your torso over your feet throughout the process.

puts exaggerated pressure on the disk and small muscles of the lower back. Taking a heavy pot off a high shelf, for example, requires caution. Stand on a stool to bring yourself closer.

When another person hands you something heavy, make sure you are near, bend your knees, and keep your back straight. These actions will help you prepare to receive the object at an altitude of three or four feet. The other person may be stronger than you are, so when you take the object, you may suffer the double jeopardy of leverage working against your lower back and a jerking that doesn't occur when you lift something off the floor.

8. Use an Abdominal Binder

This thick, corsetlike belt—the wider it is the better—wraps tightly around your body from ribs to hip bones. The shorter such a binder is, the more comfortable; however, the longer it is, the more support it can deliver. Using the Velcro, try various widths until you find the best compromise.

The support an abdominal binder provides is helpful for postural problems, discomfort after surgery, arthritis, and particularly for spondylolisthesis. An abdominal binder is worth trying if you have a disk problem. It's good for people with weak muscles, because it keeps the body straighter, making bones support more and muscles strain less. However, since an effective brace reduces the amount you use muscles and encourages dependency, exercise is a must. Use a brace to reduce pain but exercise consistently to keep up and increase your strength and improve posture. If you incorporate the better carriage into your daily life, your muscles will soon provide you with your own "subcutaneous brace."

Doctors can prescribe an abdominal binder, but even without a prescription you can try one out and then buy it at a surgical supply house or a large pharmacy.

Abdominal binders also come with special adaptations. Steel battens maintain an arch for patients who have spondylolisthesis and vertebral fractures. There are wider, specially designed abdominal binders for women, particularly for those suffering from back pain associated with pregnancy (see Chapter 13).

9. Take a Warm Bath

If you have musculoskeletal pain, sciatica, or piriformis syndrome, warm water can not only virtually eliminate gravity, but also be

---

---

soothing and relaxing, and provide relief. Spend 20 minutes submerged up to your chin in a warm (not hot) bath. You can do this two or three times a day, so long as your skin doesn't get too dry. People with multiple sclerosis shouldn't take warm baths.

10. Do Vigorous Exercise

Chronic musculoskeletal ailments that can't be attributed to a specific cause usually respond to exercise by showing an improvement of at least 30 percent within six months. Of course, a regular, vigorous, low- or no-impact exercise program must be appropriate to the individual patient and should be carefully monitored to be sure it isn't doing any harm.

Low- or no-impact exercise is best. Humans aren't built like machines that are meant to repeat the same motion again and again. What you want is exercise that produces different bodily movements and emphasizes coordination and balance. Exercise should permit one muscle group to compensate for the movement of another.

I recommend swimming, NordicTrack, proper weight lifting, Iyengar Yoga (see Chapter 3), cycling that involves arm movements, and health club exercise classes designed to avoid spine-jarring jumping around—for example, no-impact dance and step aerobics. These and Pilates (Chapter 3) are all right, but in some cases they seem to produce low back and thigh-groin pain. I believe this discomfort is caused by "too much too soon" or "too much too late." In other

---

---

words, those of a certain age should exercise enthusiastically but with care.

In general, low- or no-impact exercise is good for both nagging and intermittent pain. If slight, chronic pain doesn't get worse with exercise or is exacerbated (made worse) for only a few days, chances are good that working out will eventually control, reduce, or eliminate it.

Obviously these exercises should be done by people who can handle them. If you have a cardiac condition or osteoporosis that could make strenuous exercise risky for you, read on.

11. Do Stretching and Other Nonaerobic Exercise

Some people aren't ready and others never will be ready for vigorous exercise. But movement need not be extremely lively to be valuable. Any amount of physical exertion is better than none. Stretching (through activities such as Yoga) is one prime example of beneficial exercise that isn't necessarily vigorous. Like other nonvigorous exercise, including walking, Tai Chi (see Chapter 12), golf, and carefully moderated swimming and cycling, stretching relieves muscle spasm, postural problems, and stress. Both vigorous and nonvigorous exercise improve balance, posture, and economy of movement.

A significant amount of back pain comes from poor posture. Stretching muscles and getting them used to being of greater length and adjustable tone is useful in improving the way you walk, stand, and sit. Stretching loosens muscles that become tight when sitting at a computer, for example, and which don't relax on their own afterwards but stay tight when there is no need for them to do so. If you're experiencing a situation like this, seek this remedy, for spasm will almost invariably result.

Exercises that lengthen and strengthen muscles close to the spine are especially important for older people, who tend to hunch over and use posture to compensate for muscle weakness. People who have to make unusual gestures repetitively, like airport luggage loaders, dentists, artists and sculptors, and others who can't avoid the movements that produce pain also benefit from this type of exercise.

Once learned, the majority of the nonaerobic exercises described here can be practiced alone at home, and they have the added benefit of improving self-control, poise, and your sense of general well-being.

12. Use Chairs Effectively

Depending on how they're sat in, many different kinds of chairs are good for people with back pain. To use any chair correctly, avoid slouching, slipping down, or leaning to one side.

An upholstered chair with a seat cushion that evenly distributes the weight of sitting can help people suffering from herniated disks, piriformis syndrome, and all types of bursitis by preventing pressure in problem areas and providing support. Unupholstered straight-backed chairs bring relief to the same patients because less support and a flat seat produce better posture and better self-monitoring of weight distribution and they let the ischial bones protect the large nerves traveling through the buttocks.

13. Acquire Specialized Cushions

The advantage of special back cushions offered by pharmacies, surgical supply houses, and various catalogs is mostly that they remind the sitter to pay attention to posture in the thoracic spine, to sit up in a straight but relaxed position. A roll cushion attached to a chair back is a good example of this.

Portable and inflatable cushions meant to cover both chair seat and back are useful for spinal stenosis, radiculopathy, and musculoskeletal pains in the back.

Gel cushions that fit on the seat of a chair are thin but expensive. They can be carried like an attaché case. They're good for piriformis syndrome, coccygodynia, and muscle spasm in the buttocks and thighs.

Like shoes and abdominal binders, you should try out different cushions to see which ones are effective and comfortable.

14. Sleep on a Proper Mattress

Your mattress can be too hard, too soft, or lumpy; it might give you a backache or help you get rid of one. If it seems you're frequently "sleeping wrong" so that you wake up in the morning with a backache, the problem is probably musculoskeletal. I recommend sitting on a carpeted floor and doing a few forward bends and general whole-body stretches before going to bed for the night. If that doesn't help, get a harder mattress or a futon. If morning backache persists, wake yourself up and do the bends and stretches for a few minutes in the middle of the night.

Fifteen or twenty years ago, people preferred soft mattresses. These let the pelvis sink, flexed the hips and arched the back, sometimes causing difficulty with spinal muscles and joints. Hard mat-

---

DID YOU KNOW?

After a review of many research studies, The Agency For Health Care Policy and Research has concluded that more than four days of bed rest can actually be worse for people with backache than slowly and carefully resuming regular routines.

---

tresses came into fashion about a decade ago and are still going strong. For people who sleep on their sides, these stiff mattresses can cause problems by elevating the hips and twisting the back.

A mattress that is neither too soft nor too hard prevents the body from arching or sinking and preserves good standing posture when you're lying down. Bursitis, sacroiliac joint derangement, and arthritis require a mattress of just the right firmness. A heated water bed is ideal for trochanteric bursitis.

Replace mattresses that are more than ten years old.

15. Get Bed Rest

A herniated disk, severe musculoskeletal pain, and backache due to emotional stress can improve with bed rest. When your backache keeps you from being effective or taking pleasure in what you're doing, it's a good time to go to bed. Since the acts of getting into and out of bed are much more strenuous than they seem, it's a good idea to eat meals in bed, use a portable urinal, read or watch television there, and strictly limit time away from this restful environment. Most people feel better in less than three days. That's the proper dose of bed rest. Certainly you know you don't have the right treatment and should see the appropriate doctor if your pain hasn't improved in ten days to two weeks.

Bed rest is useless for spinal stenosis and piriformis syndrome. It makes the pain of some tumors worse, so if your pain increases after lying down for a few days, you should get up and go to a doctor.

16. Wear Loose Clothing

Whether you're wearing blue jeans or formal attire, you can be dressed in clothes so tight you can't sit down, lift, or walk properly. Your looks may be inversely proportional to the way you feel because constricting your movements with clothes prevents adaptation, adjustment, and compensations necessary to keep a back healthy. Clothes can actually change the way you walk, can change your posture, and can cause back pain.

17. Apply Ice and Heat

The time to use ice is immediately after a severe bump. Apply it as soon as possible, ideally within the first half minute after injury. Keep the ice in place for 15 minutes to half an hour if you can stand it. Ice causes blood vessels to constrict. The result is less blood in the tissues, a situation that allows the anesthetic and antiinflammatory properties of cooling to penetrate deeply. Ice might help if you suddenly find yourself in terrible pain, for example, from spasm. Though ice probably won't make a neurological problem worse, it won't help appreciably.

An electric heating pad or hot water bottle warms the outside of the body and, by a reflex mechanism actually lowers the inside temperature of the body slightly by constricting blood vessels. In other words, heat produces the same physiological effect as ice. Heat can reduce the pain due to arthritis, muscular aches and pains, and premenstrual backache. Unless heat is accompanied by massage, stretching, or ultrasound, however, the relief is no more than symptomatic.

18. Get or Give Yourself a Massage

This is an ancient and effective remedy for muscle spasm, a displaced rib, and tight or fatigued muscles, all of which can cause a great deal of back pain. If you can identify your problem as musculoskeletal (see Chapter 5), massage is definitely an appropriate remedy to try. Sometimes merely finding the muscle or muscles in question and pressing on them will relieve fierce pain.

You don't always need a person to apply the necessary pressure. Though reaching behind yourself may be difficult and can hurt, you can use a pillow or other cushion as protection and massage the aching muscle by rubbing against a doorknob or the corner of a couch. If you want a wonderful massage try lying on your back on the floor. Roll around with one or even two tennis balls under you.

In my experience, massage done by licensed therapists has been beneficial for many patients. Physical therapists use massage under the direction of physiatrists and neurologists; massage is often part of the treatment administered by chiropractors. Myofascial release is a more sophisticated form of massage based on the microanatomy of muscles. This technique, administered only by fingertips, is amazingly powerful.

Massage should not be used in cases of fracture or an active outbreak of herpes, and it can make neurological symptoms worse.

19. Change Suspicious Patterns

One of the main points I've been making all through this discussion of backache is that patients must become detectives to ferret out the causes of their own pains. If your back hurts, look for clues in your past and present. Question yourself thoroughly about what brings on the pain and what takes it away. Then, based on the ideas you've

---

TECHNIQUES TO AVOID

• Hanging   You hold on to a chinning bar and let gravity pull your weight down. This is problematical: if you're hanging by your hands, it's almost impossible to resist contracting your abdominal and back muscles, which actually compresses the spine. Hanging is too athletic and doesn't stretch any muscle.

• Lumbar Traction: This is of almost no use in most cases. A fringe benefit, however, can be the needed and enforced bed rest that lumbar traction requires.

---

come up with, experiment. Try starting or stopping exercise or other repetitive activity. Experiment safely. Change shoes, chairs, and posture. Though correcting gait irregularities usually requires physical therapy, it may be well worth having a professional examine the way you walk. It's critical to have the motivation and understanding to make the recommended changes.

20. Relax

Stress reduction through organized relaxation is helpful for loosening tight muscles and curing muscle spasm. Lie down or sit down. Think of body parts and try to relax them one by one, working upward from toes, ankles, calves, and so on. Don't neglect unseen parts: the soft and hard palates, the scalp, the eyelids, the flesh between your fingers, the anus, the hamstring muscles, and the soles of your feet. You can have someone slowly read you the following two paragraphs:

Try to individuate different sections of your back by anatomy: the left and right shoulder blades; the long latissumus dorsi muscles of the sides; the muscles of the neck; the muscles between the ribs in the front, the sides, and the back; the abdominal muscles; the muscles of the sides and lower back; and so on.

You can also relax your back by function. First release and soften the muscles from your neck that lift your shoulders. Then relax the muscles between the shoulder blades that bring them together toward your spine, the deltoids and biceps that lift your arms, the pectoralis muscles that bring your arms together in front of you, the rotator cuff muscles that bring you to the "hands up" position, the long muscles of the sides, and the muscles that arch your back and tilt your torso. Now proceed with what you've learned about the muscles of your legs and lower back.

Continue with as many symmetrical functions as you can think of. Twenty to thirty minutes is not too long for using this relaxation method. Working from within this way you often will be rewarded by figuring out exactly which muscle(s) hurt. Concentrate your thought to relax them. Breathe easily and gently, so even you can't hear yourself. It sounds paradoxical to try hard to relax, but that is what concentration is in this situation. Like any discipline, this one is difficult, but improvement comes with practice and will help you control pain.

CHAPTER 11

Medical Intervention

Whether or not you find out what's wrong, when low back pain brings you to the doctor, you're likely to walk out of the office with a prescription for a painkiller. After that the doctor's specialty has a great deal to do with the diagnostic tests you undergo and finally with your diagnosis itself. A study of 1,100 physicians illustrated the point that the field of specialization, not just the patient's symptoms and signs, influences diagnosis and treatment.

For example, orthopedists order MRIs, CT scans, and other imaging studies three times more often than other physicians. Physiatrists and neurologists rely on EMGs and electrophysiological tests. Rheumatologists favor blood work. Given these facts, it's worth your while to narrow down the field as best you can and seek the specialist most likely to recognize what you've got.

In the past, internists and primary-care physicians referred patients to the proper specialist when it was necessary. Managed care has disrupted many of the delicate referral channels, which were based on the physician's experience and judgment. So which specialist you see

and how you get to that person may be your most important decision in the process of getting better. I've discussed this in Chapter 3
and will go into it again later in this chapter, in the section on surgery.
In the meantime, it's necessary to consider what to do when you *do*
find the right doctor.

No matter what specialist recommends which test or intervention,
it's appropriate to ask questions. How well does the medicine or test
work, does it have unwanted side effects, is it worth waiting before
trying it? If you've been in pain for less than seven weeks and have no
severe neurological symptoms, imaging studies like X rays and MRIs
probably aren't necessary. Research has shown that overzealous physicians are often too early when they recommend these tests, which
have quite high rates of false-positive results.

Before you agree to any test or treatment, ask your doctor to recommend books, do your own research in the library, and if you're not
satisfied, get another opinion. As far as I am concerned, education is
preferable to medication. It lasts longer, it never expires, and there's
no such thing as an overdose. Education is invaluable for all patients,
and is second in importance only to the taking of the medical history
and the physical exam.

That said, here's an overview of some of the most commonly
used medical interventions.

Prescription Medications

Prescription-Strength Nonsteroidal Antiinflammatories   Doctors prescribe these for strain and sprain and any other causes of inflammation. These are the medicines you're likely to be given when
you've sprained a ligament or strained a muscle, and also when the
doctor doesn't know exactly what's wrong but suspects the problem
will go away by itself in time.

There are many nonsteroidal medications to choose from. Motrin
(generic name ibuprofen), Voltaren (diclofenac), and Relafen (nabu-
metone) decrease inflammation, swelling, and pain in much the same

way aspirin does. A few other drugs that work like aspirin are Naprosyn (naproxen), Clinoril (sulindac), Lodine (etodolac), and Feldene (piroxicam).

If your doctor writes you a prescription for a nonsteroidal medication, the specific drug of choice is a matter of hunch, intuition, or perhaps past experience. There's no objective way to decide which medicine will relieve your pain, but if you try one without success, don't give up; another one might work well. The chief side effect of prescription nonsteroidal antiinflammatories is gastric upset, as it is for aspirin. People who can't tolerate aspirin have the same reaction to these other medicines.

Every few months another nonsteroidal antiinflammatory medicine becomes available over the counter. I think prescription-strength dosages are not only cheaper, they're safer. You need fewer pills to supply the amount of medicine that relieves pain. Fewer pills dissolve more slowly, and you are therefore less likely to experience stomach upset.

If you do suffer gastric distress, you can take Indocin (indomethacin), a prescription medication that comes in suppository form and has no dangerous side effects in 50-milligram doses but can be problematical in higher doses. Another nonsteroidal antiinflammatory medicine called Toradol (ketorolactromethamine) can be given in injections to avoid stomach upset. Ultram (tramadol hydrochloride), a newer medicine, has fewer gastric side effects for many patients and may often be used instead of nonsteriods.

Muscle Relaxants   When physicians believe the cause of your pain is muscle spasm or muscle tightness, they naturally turn to muscle relaxants. The most common are cyclobenzaprine and carisoprodol, whose trade names are Flexeril and Soma.

Unfortunately, these compounds almost all work on the central nervous system rather than on specific muscles. Instead of releasing tension in one tight muscle, these drugs relax every muscle in your body through nonspecific sedation. Many patients who take muscle relaxants find they're seeing halos around objects or feel they're walking around on another planet.

One drug, Dantrium (dantrolene), works by weakening muscle contraction, but it, too, affects all muscles. I don't recommend dantrolene, which can cause liver damage after rather limited usage.

As a physician I prescribe muscle relaxants when I absolutely need to, but I don't like them because they're too general. Physical therapy, range-of-motion exercises, and massage are more specific to spasm and tight muscles, more physiologically appropriate, have fewer side effects, and are likely to work far longer because often they can be self-administered.

Doctors usually prescribe muscle relaxants for extreme pain they believe is temporary. These drugs aren't narcotic or addictive as they're generally used.

Tranquilizers   Valium (diazepam), Librium (chlordiazepoxide), and other tranquilizers of the type called benzodiazepines are actually more effective in loosening tight muscles than muscle-relaxant medications. I prefer them because they work better and faster (within half an hour or forty-five minutes), and most leave the body sooner. Not only do they release the patient's muscles, they help the individual sleep and they reduce anxiety. Though you won't get addicted to tranquilizers after taking them for a week-long episode of back pain, they are quite habit-forming and should be used cautiously, with medical supervision.

Antidepressants   Prozac (fluoxetine hydrochloride) and older tricyclic drugs like Elavil (amitriptyline hydrochloride) and Tofranil (imipramine hydrochloride) belong to the antidepressant group. These medications are of such significant help to people with chronic backache, they could have been introduced as painkillers. I prescribe them in very small doses (much less than is needed to medicate psychological disturbance) and find they are quite effective. They may reduce the sensation of pain by acting directly on the brain. They certainly lessen anxiety and therefore muscle tension.

Antidepressants are particularly useful for people who know what's wrong but can't correct the problem. Victims of osteoporosis, degenerative arthritis, or unhealing fractures do well with these medications. Antidepressants are often used in pain-care centers when attempts to reach a diagnosis have failed.

Often a patient has to take a tricyclic for two weeks or longer before it begins to work. If you're pregnant or have a heart or thyroid problem, don't take an antidepressant until you have corrected the problem or are a nonnursing mother.

Opiates   Morphine and heroin are natural opiates; Percocet (oxycodone and acetaminophen) and Levodromoran (levorphan) are synthetic. Both types of opiate provide excellent relief from extreme pain, for example, the pain of a vertebral body compression fracture. They work quickly when injected into a muscle and even faster when injected into a vein. They relieve pain but don't get to its cause, and of course they're extremely habit-forming. The advantage to opiates is that they buy time while healing occurs naturally or as the result of other treatment.

Patients are often worried about taking these strong drugs, but there's no cause for alarm. After taking opiates for two or three weeks you might feel an urge—a controllable desire—to continue. Unless you take opiates for six to eight weeks without a break or have a social or psychological situation that makes you vulnerable to addiction, you won't have difficulty stopping the medicine. If you're concerned, quit the pills for a day to reassure yourself, both of your control over their usage and of the indications for continuing to take them.

Needle Work

Trigger-Point Injections   Since the most common back problems are musculoskeletal, it's not surprising that muscles are the object of one of the most common treatments. Trigger-point injections are used to treat spasm, musculoskeletal pain, and piriformis syndrome. These injections into a muscle's most tender spot are done with a number of substances, alone or mixed. They take about two days to work, and here's what they do:

- Normal saline (sterile salt water) can push apart compressed or constricted structures.
- Injected steroids decrease inflammation and swelling.
- Lidocaine and other local anesthetics kill pain and immobilize local muscle fibers.

Janet Travell (John F. Kennedy's physician) and her colleague David Simons used nineteenth-century German research and their own patient studies to map out trigger points in muscles throughout the body. They found that injections into these spots relieved spasm. Now many physicians give trigger-point injections into these regions with great success. The shots are inexpensive, and though they're invasive, they rarely have unwanted side effects.

In my experience, while these injections are sometimes painful in themselves, they can seem miraculous to despairing sufferers. During an episode of back pain a patient can receive trigger-point injections frequently, getting several in a single visit to the doctor. Often this treatment works better when combined with physical therapeutic measures, for example, correcting posture or gait irregularities. You and your doctor should make sure you're not allergic to the injected substances.

When given in trigger-point injections, a new medicine, Botox (botulinum toxin type A), paralyzes muscles in spasm, eradicating pain completely within ten to twenty days. Relief lasts three to four months at least, and often up to six months. This medication is derived from the bacterium that causes botulism. It isn't dangerous, but it won't work on anyone who has been infected by or inoculated against botulism, including most veterans of the Persian Gulf War.

Epidural Injections   Doctors try using this type of injection for curing the neurological pain of sciatica, spinal stenosis, radiculopathy, and the weakness resulting from surgery, when pain has not abated. The injection of steroid with or without lidocaine, narcotics, or tranquilizer-type substances is meant to reduce inflammation, swelling, and pain. A long needle deposits the medication amongst nerve rootlets in the lumbar spinal canal. Though this injection into the lumbar spinal area is sometimes the last resort before surgery, in my experience it works only 20 to 30 percent of the time. It makes sense to have an epidural injection only if diagnostic tests show that reducing the inflammation within the spinal column is likely to relieve the pain significantly and thus interrupt a vicious cycle.

A patient came to me frustrated because she couldn't lose weight. The pain in her back made it impossible to exercise, and her inability to exercise made it impossible to control her backache. A mild narrowing of her spinal cord suggested previous vigorous exercise might have inflamed the nerves in her back. The next week an anesthesiologist administered an epidural. The outcome of the treatment was what is typically considered a success. The first injection worked for ten days, the second worked for three weeks, and the third relieved her pain for three months. During that interval she began exercising again and is now having some success keeping her back pain at bay.

Of the several hundred people I've seen who have had epidural injections, only two have complained of severe pain that they believed resulted from the procedure.

Chemonucleosis   This procedure involves visualizing the spine with a fluoroscope or other imaging technique and injecting a chemical derived from papaya (chymopapain) to dissolve part of a herniated disk that's pressing on a nerve. Injections of this type are apparently effective in 35 to 40 percent of cases. However, serious complications like chemical meningitis and a possible transverse myelitis, which kill the nervous tissue in the spinal cord, cause many physicians to think the risk is too great.

Facet Joint Injections   Facet joints between spinal vertebrae are fully as complex as knee or hip joints, and are subject to degenerative disease, inflammation, and swelling just as other joints are. Injections of lidocaine, steroid, or a mixture of the two are used to ease the pain of strain, trauma, or structural problems in these spinal structures. The shots are given directly into lumbar or other facets, or very near to the facet joint. There's no evidence of lasting benefit—facet joint injections don't reverse degenerative disease—but they do calm down transient swelling. Thus they can provide temporary relief and the opportunity to begin physical therapy and exercise.

Acupuncture   See Chapter 3 for a description of this procedure. Dry needling in which nothing is injected can be done along designated Chinese meridians or into trigger points. Needles are rotated; electrical stimulation is sometimes added. These techniques are aimed at all kinds of pain reduction.

Bursal Injection   Surprisingly often, pain in the back is due to compensation for abnormalities in the hip, knee, or ankle. Inflammation of normally small pouches of fluid can develop in the hip and knee from asymmetrical or too much sitting or walking. In my experience a local injection of steroids is successful in these cases, working for at least three months in a large percentage of patients. These injections are more effective than oral nonsteroidal medicines or any other type of medication, and they are less radical, because the medicine goes directly to, and only to, the painful spot.

I see no danger from bursal injection, even for people with diabetes, a condition that steroids might negatively affect. In the short term the lidocaine reduces the pain of the injection even though it does add fluid to an already overcrowded space. After about 48 hours the steroid begins to reduce swelling and inflammation and to decrease the volume of the fluid causing of the pain.

Diagnostic Tests

I want to emphasize once more that the history and physical exam are crucial to finding out what's wrong with your back. These two old-fashioned, low-tech rituals, performed in the doctor's office, often result in a diagnosis and should be completed before doing any of the following advanced imaging or other tests.

IMAGING STUDIES

X Ray   X rays go through muscles, nerves, and tendons to give a good visual representation of hard, dense structures—specifically bones. They're an excellent means of finding fractures and determining whether a fracture is healing properly. They're also appropriate for confirming diagnoses of spondylolisthesis, osteoporosis, dislocations, osteoarthritis, and bony tumors. Make sure you're not pregnant when having X rays of the spine.

Since a vertebral disk isn't a bone, an X ray isn't especially useful for diagnosing herniated disk. Of course, if you have an old X ray that was taken before pain began and a new one that shows vertebral bones have moved closer together, it may be reasonable to surmise that something has gone wrong with a disk.

An X ray somewhat different from the standard one is an extra long specialized X ray that can photograph the individual's spine from the neck to the hip when scoliosis (curvature of the spine) is present. Using this X ray, your physician can measure the degree of spinal curvature with a straight edge and protractor, and decide what, if any, treatment is necessary.

CT (Computerized Tomography) Scan   This test, also used to study bones, is a computer analysis of X rays taken in a machine that rotates around the body and creates a picture in cross section. All three dimensions and many different angles can be photographed. Degenerative bone disease, stenosis, and tumors show up on CT scans. This test can help diagnose a herniated disk by inference and suggestion, but isn't as good for finding that condition as an MRI (see below).

The CT scan image also shows the density of bones and is useful for diagnosing osteoporosis.

MRI (Magnetic Resonance Imaging)   A herniated disk and spinal stenosis are most easily found with this test; if you're considering surgery, an MRI is a study you should insist on having done, because it can shed light on which surgery you need.

The MRI exposes the molecules you're made of to very powerful magnetic fields (measuring 0.3 to 4 teslas), tilting them ever so slightly and sensitively detecting their positional shifts. This tints each tissue a particular shade of gray in the study, depending on the details of its structure, and produces a detailed anatomical outline.

During the imaging process you lie motionless inside a metal tube while machinery whirls and knocks. The resulting MRI is a likeness of your bony and soft tissues in all three dimensions. It shows your muscles and bursas, and gives a good outline your nerves. It's amazing how little you feel during this process, since the magnetic force is strong enough to have produced a legend about how an MRI machine pulled a 200-pound hospital worker across the room by his belt buckle.

Open MRI machines are becoming available for patients who are claustrophobic. When deciding whether to use open or closed machines, remember that the resolution (clarity) of an MRI improves in the stronger magnetic field produced by the closed-tube equipment (although software can be used to sharpen the images made with these open, low-tesla machines). Since magnetic force is used, it's essential to report any metal in your body: pacemaker, surgical clip, artificial joint, and so on. I've never heard of American dental fillings being affected.

Myelogram   Dye that will show up on films is injected into the spinal column, and then imaging studies are done. Myelograms are performed using X rays, CT scans, and MRIs. The dye highlights nerve roots as they exit the spine. Using myelograms, radiologists can take a better look at a disk that might be pressing against the "sleeve" that covers the nerve. Fluid that indicates nerve inflammation and changes in nerve density—signs of damage—is visible in a myelogram. This test also shows abnormal structures in or near the spinal cord.

A drawback to myelograms is that you might experience a temporary, harmless, but rather severe headache or backache after the completion of this test. Also, there is a very slight possibility that the injection of dye will itself injure you, causing lasting pain.

Bone Scan   Imaging studies of bones are done after the injection of a mild, safe, radioactive substance called technetium-99. This material is attracted to active bone cells, and several hours after an injection can show tumors and infections. Recent fractures are accented because of healing activity.

Gallium Scan   In a gallium scan, a radioactive "tag" that highlights inflammatory white blood cells is injected. Afterward, X-ray-like imaging depicts inflammation and overactivity in both bones and soft tissue. Though this test is used to rule out tumors and infections, it is sometimes sensitive enough to show up a very bad bruise or a significant sprain.

Sonogram   Sound waves bounce off structures in the body and, like sonar, produce a pattern on a monitor screen like the one on a television set. This test, so mild it can be used on pregnant women, detects the outlines of both hard and soft anatomical structures. It can show significant abnormalities like an aortic aneurism (a dangerous swelling in the wall of the aorta), which can cause back pain.

Thermograph   A heat-sensitive mechanism measures skin temperature on various parts of the body, producing a colorful image of the body called a thermogram. Some users claim it can pinpoint a single dermatome (a skin area served by sensory nerves coming from a single nerve root, such as L3. (See Figure 15 on page 152.)

Thermal differences are alleged to show significant variations in blood flow. Since blood heats the body, and since blood-vessel diameter is controlled by the sympathetic nervous system, the temperature of a limb is supposed to reflect proper working of the sympathetic nervous system.

People have attempted to use this technique to diagnose radiculopathy, carpal tunnel syndrome, and other entrapments. I haven't seen thermography work effectively and do not recommend it.

FUNCTIONAL TESTS

When posture causes back pain, often MRI, CT scan, and other imaging studies are normal. This fact has led to the development of a generation of computerized motion diagnostic imaging (CMDI) tests, which examine the patient's function during movement. Wearing reflective markers on anatomical trouble spots, the patient is videotaped while walking, sitting, and bending. The video signals are computerized. Then analysts can calculate the speed and torque (twisting force) of movements in any given dimension and study the path, quality, continuity, coordination, and pattern of the movement to diagnose abnormalities. Frequently these tests are used to determine a worker's ability to do a job, or eligibility to collect on an insurance claim.

I find CMDI tests time-consuming and of limited value because of the difficulties of factoring in a person's weight, size, muscle strength, and subtle compensations. I think it's preferable to observe the patient directly and in detail.

NERVE CONDUCTION TESTS

EMG (Electromyography)   EMG measures nerve conduction, velocity and strength, and the normalcy of muscle function, all important not only for pinpointing problems but in certain cases for deciding whether a patient needs surgery.

This test can definitively diagnose several conditions. It can locate a specific spot where a nerve is entrapped by identifying the place where nerve impulses slow down (for example, in the piriformis muscle) and can also diagnose neuropathy by finding several places where the speed of impulses is reduced and their strength attenuated. An EMG exam is good for showing other types of damage where muscle and nerve responses are small or irregular.

During the first part of an EMG test, your doctor will use a handheld rod attached by a wire to a larger console to administer small shocks to the skin. These minute jolts of electricity stimulate specific nerves. Then an oscilloscope, which is part of the EMG console, times and records the size and the speed of nerve impulses, measured in thousandths of a second and millionths of a volt.

In another part of the test, tiny Teflon-coated electrodes that attach to the console are inserted into muscles just below the skin (rarely causing significant pain). Then the EMG exam detects electric signals given off by muscles. For example, normal muscles are quiet at rest. But when a nerve is entrapped and no longer properly connected to a specific muscle, that muscle isn't quiet, and it gives off characteristic signals. If a group of muscles giving off such signals matches the pattern of a particular myotome (such as L4-L5), you've got a diagnosis. Your problem is a radiculopathy at L4-L5. (See Figure 15 on page 152.) Examining muscles also reveals nerve and muscle diseases, like Lou Gehrig's disease (ALS, see Chapter 9), and various myopathies (see Chapter 8).

The EMG shows how well the patient can consciously activate the muscle. A physician can see whether there has been damage that is beginning to heal or whether other nerves are starting to substitute and compensate for damaged ones. If an injured disk is pressing on a specific nerve root as it exits the spine, the electrode in the corresponding muscles will display a pattern from which a diagnosis can be made.

This test demonstrates damage to motor nerves. There is no

equivalent test for sensory nerves, whose impulses travel through the spinal cord to the brain, where they activate reflexes. For sensory nerves the H-reflex and SSEP tests (see below) are the closest equivalents of the EMG muscle exam.

H-Reflex Test   If there's something wrong in your back but the problem hasn't actually caused motor nerve damage or a problem that an EMG exam can find, this is the test of choice. It involves electrically stimulating a nerve in the back of your knee. The sensory nerve impulses travel up the sciatic nerve in spinal canal to T12 (the twelfth thoracic vertebra), where they stimulate motor cells that course right back down the same nerve to the soleus muscle in the leg. This is an electrical replica of the Achilles tendon reflex, and produces the same results. It can be used to show variations or delays in the impulses in either or both legs.

The H-Reflex test, developed by a German neurologist named Johann Hoffmann in 1917, can also diagnose a herniated disk, spinal stenosis, and other causes of low back pain and sciatica due to abnormalities occurring along the route of the reflex.

SSEPs (Somatosensory Evoked Potentials)   While an EMG reveals the conduction of motor nerve impulses, the SSEP test examines sensory impulses as they travel from body extremities to the brain. It uses two kinds of electrodes. One type emits small electric shocks that stimulate nerves; the other type—placed on parts of the skin covering the spinal cord and on the scalp over brain nerve paths— detects, times, and measures nerve impulses. The SSEP test is used for diagnosing spinal stenosis, radiculopathy, and central nervous system abnormalities caused by head injury, tumor, multiple sclerosis, and stroke.

Blood Work   Analysis of blood is often helpful in identifying rheumatological causes of low back pain. Results of blood tests can show autoimmune disease processes in which an individual's immune system attacks his or her own body. Rheumatoid arthritis, lupus erythematosis, diabetes, and kidney disease are examples. Ankylosing spondylitis and Lyme disease, which affect joints and can cause back pain indirectly, can also be diagnosed with a blood test. These tests also show Reiter's and Sjogren's syndromes, both autoimmune forms of arthritis.

Surgery

Surgery is an option for herniated disk, stenosis, spinal instability, trauma, tumors, infections, and scoliosis. Only the first three need concern us here, since a victim of trauma won't have time to sit around reading this book, tumors and infections must be treated individually, and scoliosis rarely causes pain.

The decision to have surgery is usually based on severe, disabling pain and on the results of imaging or electrodiagnostic tests. Ideally, after concluding that an operation is indicated, you would then find the right surgeon. Before the era of managed care your own doctor and word of mouth would help identify the best surgeon for you. However, it doesn't always work that way anymore. Now your doctor might send you to a surgeon whose name appears in a "provider book" to determine whether you need an operation. The surgeon, not the primary-care physician, may order and interpret diagnostic tests.

So, how to choose a surgeon? On the basis of three factors: (1) judg-

---

---

ment, (2) experience, and (3) follow-up care. As the person who might go under the knife, your job is to check the qualifications of anyone who is recommended. Interview more than one surgeon, not only about the goals of the operation and what the surgery itself will involve, but also about what you can expect before and after. Are you really the right person to undergo the proposed procedure? It's worth taking the surgeon's time to ask all your questions before you make a decision. If you opt for surgery, choose someone who has done the recommended operation at least a hundred times.

QUESTIONS TO ANSWER BEFORE HAVING SURGERY

1. How well do doctors understand which patients will benefit from the procedure?
2. How reliable are the tests that have selected me as a candidate for a particular surgery?
3. What are the chances that I am a good candidate?
4. Is the operation perfected or still experimental?
5. For how long has the operation been done?
6. Which doctors are trained to do it?
7. What is the statistical success rate of this procedure?
8. How long will recovery take?
9. Will rehabilitation be necessary?

Using the above list of questions as a guide, you and your doctor should have a thorough discussion about possible side effects and complications of surgery. Make sure you find out how long unwanted results of surgery can last and whether they can be corrected.

Of course, your physician will help you decide when to have surgery, depending on your case. Surgery for a herniated disk, for example, rarely should be done until you have tried conservative treatments for six or seven weeks. On the other hand, if major lumbar spinal instability is your problem, you should take action as soon as possible.

DISK SURGERIES

The most common reason people have back surgery is for a herniated disk accompanied by neurological signs and symptoms. Exactly when a disk is herniated enough to warrant surgery is a question surrounded by controversy. Specialists disagree because it is difficult to precisely define several of the words used to describe the condition of a ruptured disk—"bulging," "herniated," and "extruded"—not to mention identifying quirks in the individual's anatomy, the position of the disk, and the actual injury. Following are descriptions of the kinds of surgery you can have done for a slipped disk.

Microdiscectomy   This is the most common and most successful surgery for a herniated disk. Tiny instruments only 2 or 3 millimeters wide are used to make an incision in the performance of this standard, excellent procedure for removing part of a ruptured disk. If the physical exam shows disk damage, and the MRI and EMG corroborate the diagnosis, this operation has a 95 percent success rate.

After microdiscectomy (as well as following percutaneous discectomy or aspiration, discussed below), it's important to keep up your range of motion in places other than the back—ankles and knees. This doesn't threaten further injury to the disk but does help compensation and alleviate stress in those areas. Physical therapy can aid you in this, as can a sensible home exercise program. Recovery is short.

A physician friend of mine who had this surgery played tennis four days later, though he sheepishly passed when it came time to deliver his standard killer serve.

Percutaneous Discectomy, or Aspiration   A small part of the in-jured disk is sucked out or removed in other ways through a small opening. Some physicians, including myself, believe this operation should be done only if the annulus fibrosis (the disc covering) is still intact enough that it completely contains the disk. If it isn't intact, then pressures may force more disc material out after this operation, re-creating the problem.

A recent symposium on pain at the New York Academy of Medi-cine supported my reservations about these operations. Surgeons, neurologists, physiatrists, and physical therapists on the panel found that the results are often poor, because disk fragments remaining after surgery can cause nerve compression.

Percutaneous Laser Discectomy   Done with a laser rather than with an old-fashioned scalpel or suction apparatus, this operation is otherwise like the aspiration operation I just described. The laser changes the chemical and physical composition of the disk material but does not remove it. Therefore, there is the danger of nerve com-pression or irritation after this procedure. One recent study suggested the operation made no difference in 50 percent of cases.

Endoscopic Discectomy   This procedure utilizes a tiny "periscope" (called an endoscope) that is equipped with scissors and tweezers to cut off and remove disk fragments. The surgeon can see the spine through a fibroptic instrument during the operation. I think minimal disturbance of tissue around the affected disk gives this surgery an excellent chance for success, but the statistics on how well it works in practice aren't available as of this writing.

OTHER BACK SURGERIES

Laminectomy   In this operation, part of one or both laminae—the two ridges of bone at the back of each vertebra—is removed to make more space for nerve rootlets in the spinal canal (Figure 24). This good, increasingly popular surgery can be done when a bulging disk

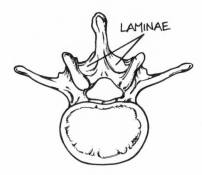

LAMINAE

Figure 24. Removing either or both of these small pieces of bone relieves pressure in the spinal canal.

reduces space and where stenosis progressively narrows the spinal canal. Laminectomy is often done on more than one vertebra; this surgical procedure, called a multiple laminectomy when done on more than one vertebra, can correct problems throughout the lumbar spine.

Occasionally removal of bone can make the spine unstable. Then this operation may be combined with spinal fusion (see below). When laminectomy and fusion are done together, the surgery is 96 percent successful.

After a multiple laminectomy, patients usually remain in bed for a couple of weeks. The need for physical therapy is individual, but some people find it useful to continue for several months.

Symptoms should be of significant intensity for three months before you decide to undergo a laminectomy, and imaging studies should confirm that you need surgery. For senior citizens experiencing pain because of spinal stenosis, I waive my usual wait-and-see approach to surgery. If that's your situation, perhaps you shouldn't put off having this excellent, highly successful operation.

Simple Fusion   Simple fusion involves a second incision at the back of the pelvis, where bone chips are removed and placed close to the unstable vertebrae. In the months following surgery, vertebral bones grow together, stabilizing but stiffening the spine.

Posterior Lumbar Interbody Fusion (PLIF)   The aim of this surgery is to re-create stability in the lower spine when it has been lost due to spondylolisthesis, fracture, traumatic injury, or infection and the victim is suffering muscular weakness and terrible pain. A long, thin rod of bone is taken from the pelvis and transplanted, usually by an orthopedic surgeon, into the spine.

Fusion alone has an 80 percent success rate and will be done more often as the population ages.

Physical Therapy

Again and again I evaluate the importance of physical therapy and come to the same conclusion. This therapeutic use of physical means is one of the most important aspects of both preventing and curing backache. Physical therapists are experts at massage, pain relief, movement analysis, exercise, and retraining.

Of course, physical therapists aren't doctors. They're not allowed to break a patient's skin, and they're not as broadly trained in the specifics of anatomy, pathology, pharmacology, and other aspects of medicine. Still, most of these health-care specialists have two or three years of hospital training. In some states a patient may bypass seeing a doctor and go directly to a physical therapist for complaints that include backache.

What follows is a more complete description of what physical therapists do.

Laying on with Hands

Cold   Studies show the use of cold is most effective during the first 20 seconds after an injury has occurred. It cools down tissue, slowing chemical reactions that produce inflammation. Blood vessels contract, which allows cold to penetrate more deeply. It's usually easier to find ice than cold-producing chemicals immediately after an injury.

In the clinic or on the playing field, cold is employed as an anesthetic and for prevention of swelling. Spray-on fluori-methane and ethyl chloride are commonly used.

Heat   Hot packs are usually placed on a painful area. The heat they deliver dilates blood vessels, increasing the flow, which unfortunately carries the warmth away before it can penetrate deeply. However, heat is pleasant and promotes relaxation. Also, the increased blood supply in the top few millimeters of skin helps heal injuries beneath the skin.

Ultrasound   This is the most effective way to deliver heat deeply into tissues. A therapist administers ultrasound with a handheld instrument that looks something like a telephone receiver. This emits piezoelectric vibrations at the rate of 800,000 to 1 million per second.

These ultrasound waves penetrate the body until they reach tissue interfaces between muscle and bone or between fat and connective tissue. There, several inches below the skin, heat may relax muscle and reduce spasm by dilating blood vessels. It has been shown that ultrasound helps speed repair of ligaments and tendons, probably by increasing blood supply.

There are variations on conventional ultrasound devices, but only the ones that deliver heat have been proven helpful. Ultrasound shouldn't be administered by anyone but licensed, experienced practitioners. Improperly used it can cause burns and tissue damage (cavitation).

Electricity   There are two forms of pain relief that electricity can provide. High-voltage impulses, delivered through stick-on disposable electrodes, cause muscles to contract tightly, pulling joints closer together. If a joint is painful because of subluxation or flaccid (flabby) muscles (as hip muscles might be after a spinal-cord injury), high-voltage electricity can improve muscle tone. Bones may come into better alignment. The beneficial effects of high-voltage electrical therapy, which can begin with the first treatment or after a number of treatments, and can last a few minutes or forever.

Low-voltage therapy is used on specific muscle fiber groups within a large muscle. The fibers contract, with a relaxing, soothing effect on the muscle as a whole. Muscle tone loosens, reducing spasm. Application of low-voltage electricity may be done with two or three pairs of electrodes that produce cross currents. Skillfully used, this method is effective for alleviating spasm and reducing pain.

LAYING ON OF HANDS

Massage   This laying on of hands (see Chapter 3) is pleasant, relaxing, and often done in conjunction with other treatments. Massage, especially some of the newer forms like myofascial release, can loosen up tight muscles, reducing spasm. Often this is critical to relieving back pain.

Mechanics of Movement   Physical therapists are trained to watch and analyze your performance of a painful movement. Breaking down an activity into its many components and examining them one by one frequently reveals a problem or pattern that is responsible for pain. Then correction and retraining can begin. After the patient understands the therapist's assessment, work can be done on altering individual parts of complex movements. Among other things, the therapist strives to teach the patient proper kinesiology (the mechanics of movement) and correct muscle balance.

With a therapist present, the patient practices reassembling a movement fully and correctly. Silly as it sounds, people are literally retaught how to walk, how to sit, and how to stand. They work on the sequence of actions involved in lifting and carrying.

Exercise   Exercising with the help of a physical therapist often involves increasing range of motion. This allows changes in the mechanics of movement to occur and is also very important in keeping people active as they age.

Physical therapists help patients with three kinds of exercises: passive, active-assisted, and active. Obviously these have different uses.

In passive exercise, you let the therapist move your body to increase range of motion, for example, in straight-leg raises meant to lengthen hamstring muscles. Though this form of movement can be extremely curative, your lack of control can also make it dangerous; injury can occur unexpectedly and suddenly.

Active-assisted exercise is when you are able to do part of an exercise by yourself but need help completing it. For example, a therapist might help you straighten and/or arch your back. By cooperating with the therapist, you can increase your strength and range of motion slowly and simultaneously.

Active exercises may be taught by therapists, but you do them on your own. Examples are push-ups, jumping jacks, and deep-knee bends and the use of machines that resist your movement. Often physical therapy begins with passive or assisted exercise designed to get you to the point of doing active exercises on your own.

Strengthening muscles is another goal of physical therapy. A number of authorities believe weakness in the muscles of the trunk is the main cause of back pain. Isotonic exercise (movement performed against a constant resistance, often with weights) is a form of active exercise that can combat muscle weakness and improve balance and coordination. Isometric exercise (done by tightening muscles but without moving) is good for strengthening when there is joint pain or a problem with posture.

Exercise can reduce spasm, regulate posture, help stabilize the spine, and relieve arthritis. It also improves the ease and safety of accomplishing a vast array of daily activities.

McKenzie Exercises   Many physical therapists rely on these, which use complex movements like side gliding and back arching, for patients suffering from a herniated disk. The goal is to identify what movements produce pain, shift the pain to the midline of your body through exercise, reduce the pain, and finally make it vanish. Then pain control techniques can be employed at home, without a therapist present.

Manual Medicine   This method combines physiologically sophisticated massage and myofascial release. There is also work with movement and exercises involving strain-counterstrain, and muscle energy techniques.

Electronic Pain Control

"Pain control" is usually reserved for situations in which diagnostic and therapeutic efforts have failed to produce relief. Attention is focused exclusively on pain reduction. Pain clinics use many different techniques and methods, but only those related to physical therapy are included here.

TENS (Transcutaneous Electrical Nerve Stimulation)   Electrodes powered by a small box reminiscent of a beeper deliver mild electrical stimulation that "fools" nerves into ignoring the pain. The masking of pain takes place because the electrical stimulation occupies many of the circuits that normally receive unpleasant sensations, leaving fewer open for perception of unpleasant feelings. TENS doesn't cure the causes of pain, but in making a person feel better this method of pain control can encourage beneficial changes in movement and posture. These gains, along with sympathetic nervous system responses, can eventually lead to permanent improvement.

Subcutaneous Devices   Electrodes are surgically placed beneath the skin in or near the spinal cord. They deliver a form of TENS if the physical therapist has found it useful. This treatment is a last resort.

Traction   This method of stretching the body to add to the degree of separation between vertebrae is usually used to ease pain in the neck or lumbar spine and to widen spaces for exiting nerves. Weighted, soft leather thongs are attached to the upper torso and either the head (for neck problems) or feet (for lumbar problems).

There are many different types of traction. Physical therapist Stanley V. Paris is well known for his cervical traction techniques, which are often done by hand. With cervical traction the idea is to achieve positive results by relieving the neck of the weight of the head (14 to 18 pounds). Depending on the situation, up to twice that amount of tension may be applied. Lumbar traction must apply at least half the person's body weight to the legs while a restraining band is placed around the chest.

In the hands of an expert, traction can help temporarily. Unless it's combined with kinesiological methods, its effects aren't long-lasting and can be harmful. Much of the "success" of traction done in the hospital is due not to weight being applied but to the patient being immobilized and therefore forced to rest for 24-hour intervals.

Mechanical Aids

Firm Braces

There are many different kinds of effective, curative braces, which are in two general categories: firm and soft. The firm braces support and guide you. They encourage the correct posture and cause pain or discomfort if you do the "wrong" thing.

Hyperextension Brace   This type of firm brace forces the back to arch and keeps weight off the front of the body. This is used for vertebral compression fractures and other conditions where leaning forward causes pain. Back braces often supplant or augment the function of muscles. Those already weak muscles get weaker the more you use these appliances, so while you're in a brace, it's important to do strengthening exercises.

Taylor and Knight Braces (for Chair Backs)   These help minimize deviations from standard posture.

Knee Braces   Knee braces, especially those with "cages" designed to keep the leg straight, can reduce functional leg-length discrepancy produced by the gait disorder called genu valgum. When the knee tilts inward to a knock-kneed position, that leg functions as if it were shorter than the other. This frequently produces back pain. (See Chapter 12 for more discussion of genu valgum.)

Ankle Braces   These firm braces are meant to increase support and reduce pain. An "air" cast, a hollow brace made stiff by inflating, cushions and supports the ankle and fills the space between it and the shoe, correcting gait irregularities that may arise from the injury and therefore preventing backache.

SOFT BRACES

Most soft braces close with Velcro and have steel ribs for support.

Abdominal Binders   These support the back (see Chapter 10). Mainly these compress the abdomen to add firmness and broad support to the torso.

Collars   Neck pain often occurs simultaneously with low back pain, and curing low back pain can help the neck. Soft collars can remind the wearer not to make jerky movements. Stiff collars put more strain on the lumbar spine by restricting and changing normal head movements.

OTHER MECHANICAL AIDS

Cane   This useful, simple tool can be used by people of all ages and for all sorts of problems and disabilities. One of its most beneficial functions is supporting the body on the side of overworked or weakened muscles. A cane is often carried on the uninjured side, improving the balancing function of the affected leg or hip.

Home Traction   This usually involves rigging up a set of pulleys with weights to relieve neck pain. I don't recommend it because it's not easy to set it up correctly and it can cause further damage to the neck.

Home Appliances   Grab bars are small secure handles attached to walls. They're exceedingly valuable in that they facilitate the use of arms to help support body weight in difficult or awkward moments, especially in the bathroom. Grab bars and other home adaptations like widening a doorway or changing the type of opening device in windows can save a great deal of pain and trouble.

Occupational Therapy

This specialty is seldom given adequate recognition. Occupational therapists do kinesiological analysis. As they study movement that causes pain, they masterfully design the most effective use of the individual's body for performing daily tasks. Unlike physical therapists, who examine posture, walking, and sitting, occupational therapists attend to everyday tasks. If putting the dishes in the dishwasher or bathing or doing the laundry causes pain, these health-care providers can help.

CHAPTER 12

Prevention Lessons

KEEPING BACKACHE AT BAY

L ow back pain, like the common cold, hits almost every adult occasionally. You pull up a stubborn weed, move the refrigerator, or for a reason you can't fathom you wake up one morning hardly able to move. With or without a doctor's ministrations, eventually you heal. You feel fine. You hope whatever made you hurt doesn't happen again.

Unfortunately, the truth is there's no way to stop it from happening, no magic pill or exercise guaranteed to keep your back healthy for your lifetime. So when you think of preventing backache, the goals of that prevention are subtle. What you're really trying to do is cut short any isolated episode of pain before it becomes chronic. It's in the space between a short-term episode and a lengthy, lingering condition that prevention takes place.

A good, realistic way to avoid chronic backache is to study effective measures for "cutting pain off at the pass," before it becomes long-lasting. The best way to do that is to look at its most common causes.

Posture

Probably poor posture is the single greatest cause of chronic low back pain.

Most of us don't have ideal posture, though if we did, it would benefit respiration and digestion as well as help avert a great many backaches. Our chairs, cars, shoes—even our clothes—aren't built to encourage good posture. Nor is good posture a value in our society.

Small children naturally start out sitting, standing, and walking erect, and at first those good habits are encouraged. But by the time most people reach their teens factors like emotion, habit, and social pressure have taken their toll. Once bad posture becomes entrenched, it doesn't change without conscious effort. That's why if you look around, you'll see that most adults slouch, arch, and lean, throwing their bodies out of balance.

CLUES

Suspect that posture explains your backache if the pain is:
- *worse at the end of the day than at the beginning;*
- *worse during the week when you sit for long periods of time at your desk than during weekends, when you both exercise and loll about;*
- *starting in the neck or upper back and spreading downward;*
- *eased by changing position;*
- *episodic—coming and going for months;*
- *sudden—beginning with a change of job, car, and so forth.*
- *utterly cured by simple massage.*

Chances are you learned while you were still in elementary school that good posture consists of standing with your ears, shoulders, hips, and ankles in one straight line. You might have walked across the room with a book balanced on the top of your head to illustrate this point and promote good posture.

TIP

For good posture, either sitting or standing, observe your upper chest—the space between your nipples and your collar bones. Open that region so that it's high and forward, without tilting your hips. The key is bringing the vertebrae closer to and keeping them parallel with your sternum (breastbone). Let the motion that brings those vertebrae toward your breastbone come from your spine between your shoulder blades. Don't do this with your breath or by throwing your shoulders back.

Proper sitting posture calls for lined-up ears, shoulders, and hips. The lowest part between your shoulder blades, your back at about the fifth to seventh thoracic vertebrae, should touch the chair behind you. Most chairs aren't designed so that's possible. Often the chair supports your ribs at the sides, just above the waist, and doesn't really provide a rest for your back.

TIP

If your chair doesn't provide thoracic support, you can use a lumbar roll pillow where you need it to bring yourself into the correct sitting posture. You can place it vertically or tie it into position on your favorite chair just below your shoulder blades.

It's crucial for correct standing posture to distribute weight properly on the feet, both side to side and front to back. Physiatrists think of the feet as bearing weight in twelve parts. Say you weigh 120 pounds. According to the clinical guidelines each foot should support half of that: 30 pounds on the heel, 5 on each toe, and 10 on the big toe. Can you achieve this ideal wearing high heels? I doubt it. But no matter what shoes you choose, it's good to attempt to stand with your weight divided this way.

T I P

*When standing, try to adjust your feet so that you are standing
with the recommended weight distribution*

Gait

The reason gait is such an important cause of low back pain is not
just that we walk so frequently, but that we're not taught to pay close
attention to what we're really doing when we walk. We go blithely
along, unaware of the many components in each step. Yet if even one
of the elements of one step consistently goes wrong, all the others
will also be thrown off, possibly with extreme consequences.

When you think about it, walking has a marvelous economy. Only
about two inches of hip bone and the muscle that attaches to the
sacrum hold up your whole body as your feet take you where you're
going. The forces exerted on that small region may be three or four
times your total weight.

C L U E S

*Gait disorders can elude identification. Pain on the sides of your
lower back and the outsides of hips should alert you to the
possibility of a problem with your gait. Back pain can arise from
the way your body's peculiarities influence your walking. Be wary if
you:*
- *have a leg-length discrepancy;*
- *have a "duck" walk;*
- *are pigeon-toed or pronate (that is, your foot or feet lean
  inward on the arch when walking).*

Walking is a series of coordinated movements. If any one of the
series of these movements goes awry, you have a gait disorder and a
potential backache. Here are some of the classic gait disorders.

Genu Valgum   One knee buckles inward when you lower your foot to the floor or pavement and put weight on it, effectively shortening that leg. You've got to raise your hip up high for the other, swinging leg to clear the floor. Your buttock, hip, and back on the buckling side will hurt. Generally, this gait disorder strikes people who are forty or older, or are overweight, have advanced arthritis, or a sports injury.

Circumduction   The leg swings out when walking because the knee doesn't bend properly. There will be pain in the buttock on the swinging side and in the lower back or sacroiliac joint on the other side.

Uncompensated Trendelenberg Gait   You limp because the weak standing leg can't support the body as you take a step. You tilt toward the strong side when your weight is on the weak side. It hurts in the lower back or the groin. The weakness that causes this disorder usually has a neurological cause, such as radiculopathy or spinal-cord injury.

Compensated Trendelenberg Gait   The upper part of the body swings out over the weak leg in an adaptation. You unwittingly bring your weight over the weak leg when you are supporting your weight with it during walking. It hurts in the lumbar spine.

Footslapping   This is opposite of pointing your toe. During walking, the forefoot slaps the pavement instead of connecting smoothly with it. This gait disorder arises from muscle weakness due to multiple sclerosis, radiculopathy, or stroke. Adapting to the problem of footslapping often causes pain in the quadraceps or in the backs of thighs. It can also lead to unequal step size (see below).

Unequal Step Size   This gait problem can cause pain in the lower back or pelvis. It comes about through loss of range of motion, problems in weight-bearing joints or asymmetrical weakness.

Loss of Range of Motion in Hip, Knee, or Ankle   These are major but subtle sources of back pain. Range of motion is limited by bad habits, arthritis, injury, or disuse. Loss of range of motion can be at the bottom of many different gait disorders, which a trained specialist can identify by watching you walk. A large number of gait disorders are easily cured.

T I P

A simple aid to adaptation, an orthotic or heel lift, often worn inside a shoe or beneath the clothing, can correct a gait disorder. Physical therapists give gait training as well as exercises to increase range of motion.

Exercise

But isn't exercise the best prevention for back pain? Yes, depending . . . I don't advise exercise that is simply repetitive. Properly varied, exercise is invaluable. However, I take a dim view of the misuse of health clubs. At least in Henry Ford's assembly lines, they paid you. Now some people rush to the health club where they pull the same lever all day to pump up their muscles or they run on the treadmill with the same movements to get aerobic exercise. The biggest drawback to repetitive exercise is that it doesn't allow us to do what we do best—adapt.

T I P

Don't rely on one type of exercise; treat the gym as a smorgasbord. A variety of exercises done with attention to back safety is best for maintaining a healthy back.

The drawback to doing repetitive exercise is that we are cunning animals. After tiring the muscles of the arms or legs by repeating the same action, we are likely to substitute the stronger muscles and levers of our backs. This, of course, leaves us open to injury. Also, many exercises and devices designed to work specific muscles like the biceps put your back in mechanical jeopardy. The excellent trainers many health clubs provide can help you design a varied, safe exercise program.

There's every reason to believe the research that says you've got to get your heart beating fast for 15 or 20 minutes a day at least three times a week. But there are excellent orthopedic, kinesiological, and physiological reasons for altering your activity in the course of the exercise. I recommend exercising in a way that's called cross training. Say you run for five minutes, then do some pushups and jumping jacks, and finally swim; or after a game of tennis you lift weights and stretch. Even if the repetitive nature of one or more of these activities were harmful in itself, varying your actions and not getting into a rut saves your muscle, cartilage, joint capsule, and bone. And your back!

Exercise can cause back pain, but exercise is also one of the great ways of staving off that very pain and keeping it from becoming chronic.

T I P

Regular exercise has been proven to limit the number of episodes of back pain, to shorten them, and to reduce their severity. Some people find they must exercise to prevent back pain.

Here's why you need exercise:

• Stronger muscles support and hold the body together, preventing problems with ligaments, disks, and joint capsules and defending against poor leverage.

• Increased flexibility distributes strain over a larger area and reduces the possibility of injury.

• Increased range of motion near a fragile, painful joint allows for compensation to take place.

T I P

Pay attention to your movements during any type of exercise; be aware of and stop anything that causes more than a mild twinge. You don't want progressive discomfort that comes from anything other than pure fatigue.

RECOMMENDED EXERCISES

Swimming   The fluid movements of swimming are safe because the water both buoys you up and slows you down, preventing awkward, injurious movement. The backstroke, crawl, and breaststroke are good for increasing range of motion. The sidestroke is least dangerous for your back. Swimming is aerobic, but unlike some other aerobic exercise it can't help you lose weight. Don't swim for three months after a lumbar spine fracture has healed.

Yoga   Like swimming but without water, Yoga involves slow, controlled movements. You can mix standing, sitting, lying down and inverted poses. Yoga is good for balance, strength, flexibility, endurance, and alertness. It's not repetitive and need not be weight-bearing. The Yoga student slowly and self-consciously tries to increase range of motion and relax. I find the Iyengar Yoga method, which has associations of certified teachers in many cities throughout the world, the most anatomically sophisticated.

Tai Chi   This moving exercise system originated in ancient China and is popular today, both here and abroad. Concentration and focus are necessary to perform a specific sequence of movements. These movements "ground" the participant, helping to balance and increase leg strength. The result is better body awareness and an opportunity for relaxation of specific tension spots. If exercises are done correctly, they are good for body alignment (posture) and provide both direct and indirect help for back pain. Tai Chi should be taught by certified instructors. For more information, contact the Tai Chi Foundation in Reston, Virginia.

Weight Control

Extra weight increases stress on the body and causes imbalance, which raise the odds for an episode of back pain and increases the stakes for the severity and duration of the pain. There's a natural tendency for people to sit more, become less active, lose strength, and gain weight as they approach middle age. Yet it's these grown-ups who are the most likely to lift and carry heavy objects, including bicycles, suitcases, and overly full stomachs.

When you're overweight, your center of gravity moves from where it's supposed to be (in your spine near vertebra S2) to a spot closer to the front of your pelvis. Your back compensates by arching more. The heavier you are, the more likely your back is to hurt. When you're walking, the extra weight puts pressure on your back and sacrum. Added padding on your buttocks can squeeze into the spaces between bones that are needed to isolate and protect nerves. All this puts you at risk for:

- herniated disk;
- muscle strain and sprain;
- facet joint problems;
- painful feet;
- temporarily pinched nerves, such as piriformis syndrome.

T I P

Limit caloric intake, and you will inevitably shed pounds. (See Chapter 10 for a simple, effective dieting technique.)

While lifting sedated patients, a hospital aide who worked in the operating room and was 30 pounds overweight continually reinjured himself. He tried a broad belt used by weight lifters and experimented with other contraptions, but nothing worked. I suggested he come closer to the patients he had to lift and lose weight if he didn't want to hurt himself. One day my words clicked. Without saying anything, he began going to meetings at Weight Watchers. Eventually he did so well he got rid of his built-in extender. Now he can work double shifts, and his back is perfect.

Unlike this ambitious gentleman, many of my patients feel they can't lose the weight that is absolutely crucial to lose in order to have a healthy back. It seems impossible to them that they will ever get into the statistical category recommended for their age, height, and gender. When I suggest a diet, these people generally say the same thing: "I hardly eat at all, but I gain weight anyway."

"You may not be aware of every morsel you're eating," I reply.

"I know very well what I eat" is the typical rejoinder.

When given a notebook and asked to write down each bite they take and show me the results, these patients rarely do. "Today was different," is one reason they give me. Or, "I did eat the leftovers, but that didn't amount to anything."

T I P

If you're carrying extra pounds and want to become thinner, you can wear an abdominal binder, which will physically pull in your stomach and make you slightly more aware of what you put in it. Some physicians, for example Dr. Richard Bernstein of Mamaroneck, New York, are expert at producing weight loss by treating patients with medications used to correct obsessive-compulsive disorders.

Stress

PHYSICAL STRESS

Physical tension, no matter what its source, makes you a candidate for back pain. Sometimes muscles tighten in response to the generalized fatigue that comes from lack of sleep; other times they tense because they are overworked. Muscles that are too taut can impair balance and coordination, or make a person vulnerable to spasm or back injury.

T I P

Lighten up. Your purse, briefcase, or backpack may weigh five times what it needs to. If so, your back may suffer. Sometimes it's sound to buy two of something. For example, avoid having to stop at the doctor's office on your way from your home to your office by buying a second copy of the heavy reference book you've been lugging to and fro.

T I P

Eat well. One antidote to physical stress is a healthy, simple diet consisting of as many fresh fruits and vegetables as possible. Forget the fried, processed foods your body has to work so hard to digest.

T I P

Have fun. This prescription applies to both physical and emotional stress. When you're overtired and worried, when the deadlines loom, take a break. Do what you enjoy, whether it's strolling in the park or peeling paint off the side of a boat. It's often more beneficial to do something that gives you pleasure than it is to lie down, close your eyes, and sleep.

EMOTIONAL STRESS

There's no question that emotional stress has an effect on back pain. It can lead to physical signs like clenching the teeth, tapping the feet, and general stiffness. Research has proven that there can be a difficult emotional component even to happy events like going on a honeymoon.

When you are experiencing emotional distress, your posture changes. The way you sit, stand, and move is less likely to be balanced and symmetrical. You may not be standing on your feet in the correct weight distribution. You may be out of synch with your center of gravity. Of course, all this makes injury more likely. Stress causes people to become irritable, to act in an abrupt or impetuous way that also leaves them open to physical mishaps.

Another result of anxiety and tension is a loss of self-esteem. Worried, overworked, strained people have less motivation and energy for taking good care of themselves. A person in this condition might slam a car door rather than shut it carefully, might not bend his or her knees when picking up a heavy object, and might not muster up the discipline for regular physical exercise.

Dr. John Sarnow, a professor of rehabilitation at New York University's School of Medicine and attending physician at the Howard A. Rusk Institute of Rehabilitation, has made significant inroads into back pain by helping patients work on stress, which generates a vicious cycle for many people who have chronic backache. Stress and backache are like the chicken and the egg. For some there's no answer to the question of which came first and caused the other.

T I P

Do something you enjoy. Of course, the best way to deal with stress is to figure out what's causing it and take action to correct the problem. But you might not be able to do anything about the state of your finances, your final exams, or a relationship difficulty. Whether or not you can eliminate the cause of your stress, my advice is the same. Have fun. Relax. Go to the movies, swim, take a walk.

What I do in stressful times is Yoga, but any mild, comfortable activity will do you good. Try Tai Chi or sit quietly and meditate. A change in your normal routine is sometimes enough to break a cycle of tension. Dr. Sarnow's methods have helped many.

Back Schools and Education

Many of my patients have asked my opinion of the back schools sprinkled across the country. Back schools offer group sessions that are led by physiologists, physical therapists, or physicians, and are intended to teach patients how to raise their level of functioning and avoid future injury.

A back school may have some value for mild, nagging, chronic backache, or for people whose backache is related to occupation. Exercises and pointers are disseminated to large groups in back schools, and some people benefit from the group environment. Also, your fellow sufferers make up a peer pressure group to help you follow the suggestion that it's better to grin and bear it than to complain.

While back schools may be all right for some individuals, they have their disadvantages. For one thing, classes may be taught by nonexperts. You receive little or no individual attention, so it's easy to get lost in the group.

I don't recommend back schools for people with new or severe pain.

I think reading is generally a more effective educational tool than a back school. There's a wealth of educational material available for people with backache. Sorting through the newsletters and the popular books with their varied approaches is something like searching for the right practitioner. Check the authors' credentials and affiliations, and choose what you read according to your own individual needs. Your doctor can recommend books and may also have extremely helpful printed handouts available.

CHAPTER 13

Sex and Pregnancy

T hough back pain is more prevalent during pregnancy than it is at other times, in the natural course of events, sex proceeds pregnancy. So it seems logical to start with a discussion of lovemaking and low back pain—how the two conflict and how that conflict can be resolved.

Sex

Most experts agree that backache can be a real drawback to the kind of intimacy we enjoy and even require. Nor is there much controversy about the primal, characteristic movements of sex. These movements, seen throughout the animal kingdom, are painful for both men and women who are suffering from any one of a variety of common back ailments. The primitive sexual motions of thrusting and pulling back can make existing pain worse, and in some cases can cause pain where before there was none.

Fortunately, there is a great deal you can do to prevent both episodic and chronic back pain from putting a significant crimp in your sex life.

COMMUNICATE AND PLAN

Remember, you're not alone with your back pain. You have it, but your lover also has a partner who has it. No matter how difficult, it's worth discussing what does and what doesn't hurt—before, during, and after sex. If two people can talk about and orchestrate their sexual union for their mutual pleasure in spite of backache, they will have achieved more intimacy than many couples who never experience a twinge. Your ultimate goal in sex, after all, is happiness and satisfaction for both partners.

Of course pain itself makes a person tense. The fear of pain is also an important source of emotional distress that can inhibit sexual desire. Both backache and the anticipation of it can turn people off so that they just don't want to or can't get involved in sex at all. A woman may be afraid to begin foreplay that will end in intercourse, which may be painful for her back; if she does start the process and then succeeds in having intercourse, tension may prevent her from having an orgasm. Men sometimes find that the idea of pain, as well as actual discomfort, prevents them from attaining an erection.

POSITIONS

In general, nature allows couples with back pain (in one or both partners) to get along and solve their sexual problems. Of course, this is a highly individual subject, not just with regard to hurt backs and human anatomy, but also when it comes to personal preference, physical and emotional style, and even furniture. Nevertheless, there are some standard ways you can set the stage for having a pleasurable sexual experience in spite of backache.

Dos

There are several positions I can recommend:

• Spoon Position   Whether one or both partners has back pain, physicians and other health-care providers in many cultures almost universally recommend the spoon position for comfort during sexual intercourse. This position involves both partners lying on their sides, facing the same direction, knees bent, the man nestled against the woman from behind (Figure 25).

• Reversed Missionary Position   The standard missionary position with the man on top of the woman may activate or cause back pain. Regardless of whether man or woman or both are suffering from back pain, I advise having sex with the woman on the top and the man on the bottom. And remember, the man must keep his legs bent.

• Seated   The right chair can support a man's painful back while the woman sits, facing him, on his lap.

No matter what position you and your partner find best, take it easy. Extreme, abrupt, overly vigorous movements can bring on pain. Make sure you control your movements, and that they stay mild and gentle.

Keep yourself physically fit by exercising. Pay attention to strength-

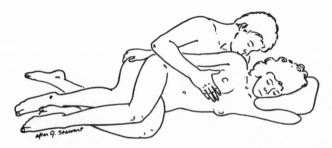

Figure 25.   The spoon position—good for either party, therefore good for both.

ening and maintaining the tone of muscles that support the spine, both in the back itself and in the abdomen.

Partners who want an active sex life in spite of back pain need to use imagination to find solutions to their problems. Without going into every detail, I can make a few suggestions: Consider unusual environments for sexual activity; for example, a water-filled bathtub or hot tub can provide some buoyancy and reduce pressure on delicate spines. Try sexual activities that don't involve traditional intercourse.

Don'ts

If you are in extreme pain due to spasm or another problem, it isn't appropriate to attempt to have sexual intercourse. Wait until 48 hours after severe pain has abated to make love.

Never increase pressure on the iliopsoas muscles, which attach to the inner thigh on one end and on the other end to lumbar vertebrae. To avoid stretching these muscles

- keep knees bent at all times;
- don't arch your back more than necessary;
- don't lie flat on your back with your legs straight out.

Dealing with Piriformis Syndrome

Women who suffer from sciatica due to piriformis syndrome often have a condition called dyspareunia. They experience sharp, severe vaginal pain during penetration. The solution is a pillow placed under the buttock on the affected side. This causes most of the action to occur on the normal side and avoids irritating the sciatic nerve.

Sex after Surgery

All the information about sex and backache in this chapter applies to your situation if you've just had surgery. Whatever the action or movement, if it increases pain, stop. After surgery, it's a good idea to start with sensate focus (which I will discuss shortly) and progress gradually.

GOOD NEWS ABOUT SEX AND BACK PAIN

Even relatively minor bouts of back pain with musculoskeletal origins can lay you up and lay you low. However, of and in itself, sex is undeniably an exercise. If you're sure your back pain isn't caused by a neurological or structural instability (from spondolisthesis, for example, or from fracture), engaging in gentle, slow lovemaking may actually help you heal faster. And this kind of sexual activity may also contribute to the maintenance of a healthy back.

SENSATE FOCUS

If all else fails, the technique of sensate focus is valuable for people whose back pain is negatively affecting their sex lives. It's particularly beneficial for people with chronic back problems and for patients recovering from surgery. Not only does it help revive a couple's physical relationship, it often provides the bonus of improving two people's ability to communicate and to give and receive affection.

The idea of sensate focus is to work up to having sexual intercourse gradually, over time. Begin by making a date—the first of six—with your partner. Set aside 45 minutes or an hour when there's nothing else happening. Turn off the phone, make sure the kids are safely asleep, or go away for the night. Then change into comfortable or night clothing and take to your bed.

Once in bed, your goal is to offer and accept pleasure without producing pain. Sex is not on the menu. I advise couples to talk, to massage each other gently, to snuggle, to relax. Knowing ahead of time that this togetherness is just that—not preparation for actual intercourse—helps relieve fear, tension, and inhibition.

Sensual activities progress, but slowly, during each of the half-dozen romantic encounters. Pleasure, not sex, is the object. Each partner should take into consideration and act on feedback from the other. If one approach doesn't work or produces pain, find another. The process of exchanging affection is a creative one, and people get better at it with practice.

I advise partners to hold off trying to have sex until the seventh sensate focus session. Even then intercourse need not be the primary aim. A couple's level of sexual "achievement" is often higher when the partners are careful not to expect too much.

Pregnancy

Why Pain Strikes

Temporary backache, sometimes severe, strikes many women at the moment they are giving birth, and after having a baby. As many as 54 percent of women suffer low back pain at some point during a pregnancy, and a large number have intermittent aches for the whole nine months. The backache common during a pregnancy can usually be prevented or substantially relieved.

This pain has several well-known causes.

Weight Gain   Added weight puts a strain on muscles. The placement of that weight and its uneven distribution change a woman's center of gravity (see Chapter 12), leading to poor posture. In order to maintain balance she arches her back. The result is nagging low back pain and spasm in overworked muscles.

An obvious, at least partial, solution to the problem of weight gain is to limit the pounds you put on. Discuss how much weight you ought to add with your obstetrician, and follow a sensible diet so that you don't exceed what's recommended.

Postural Changes   Just opposing gravity by staying upright puts immense pressure on the pregnant woman's back muscles. It has been estimated that during the last three months of pregnancy, a woman walks around as though she were carrying 25 percent more weight than the sum of herself and the baby. In other words, a woman who normally weighs 100 pounds and has gained 20 pounds since conception is subject to forces equivalent to an extra 50 pounds.

Weakness   As a woman's abdomen swells to make room for the baby during pregnancy, the muscles stretch. The abdominal muscles lose strength, and in many women they become downright weak. Dr. Avital Fast, Chairman of the Department of Rehabilitation at the Albert Einstein College of Medicine in New York, has found that only 21 of 164 women he tested could do a single push-up during the last trimester of pregnancy.

Hormonal Changes   To prepare an expectant mother's pubic bones and sacroiliac joints for the baby's journey through the birth canal, the placenta manufactures and releases a hormone called relaxin. This substance loosens the ligaments that cross exactly those joints stressed by the weight of the fetus. These joints must bear the extra weight of late pregnancy too. The weight forces them apart, producing pain. Then the woman often compensates for that pain with further postural adaptation, making it even worse.

Increased Blood Volume   During pregnancy the amount of blood in a woman's body increases. This can distend already enlarged pelvic veins, causing pelvic congestion syndrome (see Chapter 9). Blood also collects in Batson's plexus—the network of veins inside the spinal column. Congestion can arise in that narrow bony space. The result is pressure against nerve roots, which brings about pain like that of spinal stenosis and radiculopathy.

To reduce the pain caused by pelvic congestion syndrome, bricks can be placed under the legs at the foot of the bed so that the expectant mother is lying in a position that allows blood to drain toward the head. Inverted Yoga positions (for example, head-and-shoulder stands), done with the supervision of an experienced practitioner, also accomplish this. Also useful is a slant board, a wedge-shaped mat a woman can lie down on so that her head is lower than her feet. If you have problems with your lungs or heart, consult your obstetrician before attempting to use any of these methods.

Sleep Difficulties   Pregnant women often sleep poorly, especially during the last trimester. This not only deprives them of the REM (rapid eye movement) sleep associated with creative thinking and problem solving, it makes them irritable and accident-prone.

NIGHT OR DAY

You can sometimes determine the nature of your pain and how to treat it by when it occurs.

Daytime
Back pain. Musculoskeletal back pain that gets worse with particular movements and better with rest is common in pregnant women.

The aches, pains, and muscle strains caused by daily activity should

abate when you sit down comfortably or relax in bed. Postural training and strengthening exercise, braces, massage, myofascial release,
ultrasound, and for joint pain dry needling can also help for much
longer.

Dry needling is unlike acupuncture. Acupuncture needles are inserted along predetermined meridians to produce anesthesia. Dry
needling, done with ordinary medical injection needles, relieves pain
through mechanical disruption of muscular or connective tissue. It
can ease pain resulting from calcium deposits, for example, or from
muscle spasm.

Hip pain. Again, if this occurs with activity, the cause is probably
musculoskeletal. Relieve this discomfort by changing position or
moving to a more comfortable chair. Work on both sitting and standing posture.

If hip pain occurs only with activity, you could have temporary osteoporosis, a condition believed to be related to calcium metabolism
and hormonal changes in pregnancy. This almost always disappears
within a few months after the pregnancy ends.

Pelvic pain. You should feel better when sitting comfortably with
your legs and feet up if the pain has its origins in weight gain, hormonal changes, or weakness in your abdominal muscles. Change position frequently. Use a physical therapist to try to improve your
posture. Do isometric exercises (see Chapter 11). For relief of severe
pain, a sacroiliac belt designed for use during pregnancy might do
some good. A cane helps you support yourself from above and can
provide a great deal of relief.

Nighttime

Back pain at night is likely to have vascular origins and to keep you
from getting sufficient REM sleep. The combination of lying on your
back, the weight of the baby, and increased blood volume causes
pressure against the vena cava, the large vein that collects blood from
all over the pelvis and spinal cord and returns it to the heart. This increases congestion and discomfort. Often just turning over provides
quick and substantial relief. The inverted postures described earlier
on page 262 can also reduce discomfort. Place pillows between your

legs to reduce pressure and near your back to prevent you from assuming the recumbent position that caused the difficulty in the first place.

These remedies work well for nighttime pelvic pain.

PAIN ALL THE TIME

Here are descriptions of back symptoms that need the attention of a doctor who can make a diagnosis:

Pain that Goes Down the Leg with Weakness or Numbness   An EMG (see Chapter 11) is safe for pregnant women and can pinpoint the source of neurological symptoms.

Severe Pain Very Low in Back   There are several ways to rule out sacroiliac joint derangement (see Chapter 9) during a simple office physical exam. Unfortunately not all obstetricians are conversant with these diagnostic methods. A physiatrist or an osteopath can both find and treat this condition without endangering the baby. You can wear the specialized sacroiliac joint brace described above. Physical therapy with muscle energy and strain/counterstrain techniques can bring relief.

Note: These suggestions assume that you are nowhere near your due date and are not experiencing back labor.

Exquisite Pain   In spite of postural changes during pregnancy and other risk factors, pregnant women are no more vulnerable to herniated disks than the rest of the population. However, it's not impossible. A herniated disk could be difficult to diagnose, because X rays are not indicated for pregnant women, especially not in the first and last trimester. Nor have MRIs been approved as safe for the mother and baby. Few medicines are considered safe. An EMG and a good physical exam are best for diagnosing a herniated disk. Should your doctor decide a disk problem is responsible for the pain, conservative measures—bed rest and physical therapy including McKenzie exercises—should help.

Hip Pain that Doesn't Go Away with Rest   In rare cases this pain may be caused by avascular necrosis, which is quite serious and should be diagnosed and treated immediately. See an orthopedic surgeon.

PIRIFORMIS SYNDROME

In some cases, the added weight of the baby causes the piriformis muscle in the middle of the buttock to put pressure on the sciatic nerve. The piriformis muscle originates on both sides of the sacroiliac joint and tightens with pelvic instability and sacroiliac joint derangement. This produces buttock pain that is worse when sitting down. If you have piriformis syndrome, you can diagnose yourself. (See Figure 18, page 168.)

Pressing on the muscle in the mid-buttock will produce the pain. Also, lying on your "good" side and bringing the thigh on the affected side up so the hip is flexed to 90 degrees will cause the pain. See a physiatrist. The solution to the problem is ultrasound and stretching exercises, dry needling, and wearing a pelvic instability belt.

SAFE MEDICAL INTERVENTIONS

When backache interferes with daily activities, it's often necessary to take action. Of course, the problem is that many medicines and procedures could affect the well-being of the developing baby. Still, there are a number of harmless medical interventions worth trying.

Physical Therapy   This is the mainstay of dealing with back problems during pregnancy. Since most pregnancy-related backache is due to posture and muscle problems, the medical specialist most likely to be of use is a physiatrist, who directs courses of physical therapy. You may need the movement analysis and correction and other physical therapy outlined in Chapter 11.

The pregnant woman or new mother can learn all over again how to sit, stand, walk, and even lie in bed. Both isotonic and isometric exercises can contribute to readapting the spine, strengthening muscles, and improving posture.

Dry Needling   The injection of steroids or lidocaine may be considered dangerous during pregnancy. This rules out trigger-point injections. Still, dry needling can very effectively relieve pain and is completely safe.

Glossary

allodynia [al-oh-DINN-ee-a] When a generally nonpainful stimulus (for example, cloth against skin) is painful.

asymmetrical Not occurring in the same place on both sides of the body.

bursas Small fluid-filled pouches that protect muscles, tendons, and bones near joints.

bursitis Painful inflammation of a bursa.

carpal tunnel syndrome Painful compression of the median nerve at the wrist, causing weakness and numbness in the hand.

cervical Referring to the part of the spine between the head and the first rib (C1 through C7).

coccygodynia [COCK-sih-go-DINN-ee-a] Damage to or breakage of the coccyx (tailbone).

CT (computerized tomography) scan Computerized X-ray procedure that gives cross-sectional pictures of the body; especially revealing of problems in bones.

diagnosis The cause of illness, disease, or injury that can produce signs and symptoms.

disk The rubbery structure, shaped like a hockey puck, that separates one spinal vertebra from another, adding flexibility to the spine.

electromyography (EMG) A diagnostic test used by physicians to determine whether nerves or muscles are damaged, and if so, where, and often why.

facet joints Tiny joints that link spinal vertebrae; each vertebra has four facets, two above and two below.

fusion A surgical procedure in which bone fragments from elsewhere in the skeleton are placed between spinal bones, with the goal of having them grow together after surgery to form a solid unit.

herniated disk The damaged or broken surface of the disk that separates spinal vertebrae; also called "slipped disk," "ruptured disk," and "herniated nucleus pulposus (HNP)."

kinesiology [kin-eez-ee-OLL-ogy]   he study of the physical aspects of movement: muscles, bones, coordination, and gravity.

laminectomy A surgical procedure to remove the back part of the vertebral arch on one or both sides of the spine, sometimes at multiple levels.

ligaments Leathery strands of connective tissue between one bone and another.

lumbar Referring to the five vertebrae between the ribs and the sacrum (L1 through L5).

lumbosacral Referring to the lumbar spine plus the sacrum (L1 through L5 and S1 through S5).

microsurgery The use of very small instruments to lessen the trauma of surgery, usually for removal of precise portions of damaged disk or bone.

musculoskeletal Referring to structures that include muscles, tendons, ligaments, bones, and joints.

myelogram A diagnostic imaging test done after the injection of a radiopaque substance into the spinal space.

myofascial [my-oh-FASH-al] **release** Fingertip manipulation to loosen connective tissue.

nerve bundles of nerve fibers (see below), usually outside the spinal cord and brain.

nerve entrapment When a nerve is compressed or "pinched" in a narrow space, causing discomfort or pain and temporary or permanent injury.

nerve fiber A small number of specialized cells transmitting impulses that convey information about sensations or cause movement.

nerve roots Paired bundles of nerve fibers exiting the spinal cord between each two vertebrae, for example, at right L4 and left L4; soon after leaving the spinal cord, nerve roots combine and their fibers regroup into individual nerves.

orthopedist A physician specializing in problems of the form and function of bones, joints, and muscles.

osteoarthritis Progressive degeneration of joints due to normal or abnormal wear and tear.

physiatrist [phizz-ee-AY-trist] A physician specializing in physical diagnoses, who uses hands-on means of treatment, with emphasis on restoring lost function. Also called a "doctor of physical medicine and rehabilitation."

piriformis syndrome Compression of the sciatic nerve by the piriformis muscle in the buttock.

radiculopathy [rah-DIK-yoo-LOPP-uh-thee] A compression or pinching of a spinal nerve root.

reflex An involuntary movement brought about when nerves activate a muscle in response to a stimulus applied to a sensory nerve.

reflex sympathetic dystrophy A painful imbalance arising from the autonomic nervous system and usually affecting an arm or leg.

ruptured disk See "herniated disk."

S and L Abbreviations for "sacral" and "lumbar." Physicians use these abbreviations (along with T for "thoracic" and C for "cervical") to refer to specific spinal locations. They are usually associated with numbers that designate particular vertebrae; for example, C3 is the third cervical vertebra. Thoracic vertebrae are numbered from 1 to 12, lumbar from 1 to 5, sacral from 1 to 5, and cervical from 1 to 7.

sacroiliac joint derangement Misalignment of the sacrum with respect to the iliac bones.

sacrum A large central bone supporting the entire spinal column and wedged between the two sides of the pelvis.

sciatica Pain or discomfort that travels down the buttock and leg in the pattern and path of the sciatic nerve, the body's largest nerve.

scoliosis Curvature of the spine, which usually causes no back pain.

sign A result of a diagnostic test; an objective indication of injury or disease (contrast with "symptom").

slipped disk See "herniated disk."

spasm A painful, prolonged (minutes to days), involuntary muscle contraction brought on by a neurological condition.

spasticity An abrupt, exaggerated, easily triggered reflex usually brought on by a neurological condition.

spinal stenosis A narrowing of the inside of the spinal column.

sprain When fibers of a ligament or tendon are partially or completely torn.

steroids Prescription medications that calm inflammation by imitating or replicating natural adrenal compounds.

strain When a muscle, tendon, or ligament is "pulled" or otherwise made to work beyond its usual range, sometimes producing a little bleeding in the muscle.

subluxation A minor misalignment of bones in a joint.

symmetrical Occurring in the same place on both sides of the body.

symptom Something you feel, like pain or tingling; a subjective indication (contrast with "sign").

symptom of an illness.

tendon A strong, leathery strand of tissue connecting a muscle to a bone or to another muscle.

TENS (transcutaneous electrical nerve stimulation) A battery-powered device that uses mild electrical stimuli to mask pain.

thoracic Referring to the part of the body enclosed by the ribs, including the spine from T1 through T12.

vascular Having to do with arteries, veins, and the lymphatic system.

vertebrae The bony segments of the spinal column.

Bibliography

Agency for Health Care Policy and Research. *Acute Low Back Problems in Adults.* Clinical Practice Guideline no. 14. Rockville, Md., 1994, Publication 95-0642.

Barrett, John, and Douglas N. Golding. *The Practical Treatment of Backache and Sciatica.* MIT Press, Boston, 1984.

Benson, Herbert, with Miriam Klipper. *The Relaxation Response.* New York, Avon Books, 1974.

Cailliet, Renee. *Soft Tissue Pain and Disability.* F. A. Davis, Philadelphia, 1977.

Cherkin, Daniel, Richard Deyo, Kimberly Wheeler, and Marcia Cole. "Physician Variation in Diagnostic Testing for Low Back Pain," *Arthritis & Rheumatism,* vol. 37, no. 1 (January 1994), pp. 15–22.

Cohen, J. E., et al. "Group Education Interventions for People with Low Back Pain: An Overview of the Literature," *Spine,* vol. 19 (June 1, 1994), pp. 1214–1222.

Chu-Legraff, Q. et al. "Hukebein Specifies Aspects of CNS Precursor Identity Required for Motorneuron Axon Pathfinding," *Neuron,* vol. 15, (November 1995), pp. 1041–1051.

Dellon, A. L., S. E. Mackinnon, and P. M. Crosby. "Reliability of Two-Point Discrimination Measurements," *Journal of Hand Surgery*, vol. 12A, no. 5 (1987), p. 5.

Doty, James R., and Setti S. Rengachary, (eds.). *Surgical Disorders of the Sacrum*. Thieme Medical Publishers, New York, 1994.

Dimaggio, A., and V. Mooney, "The McKenzie Program: Exercise against Back Pain," *Journal of Musculoskeletal Medicine*, vol. 4 (1994), pp. 63–73.

Desforges, Jane F. "Clinical Use of Bone Densitometry," *New England Journal of Medicine*, vol. 324, no. 16, (April 18, 1991), pp. 1105–1109.

Endresen, E. H. "Pelvic Pain and Low Back Pain in Pregnant Women—An Epidemiological Study," *Scandinavian Journal of Rheumatology*, vol. 24 (1995), pp. 135–131.

Fast, Avital. "Low Back Disorders: Conservative Management," *Archives of Physical Medicine and Rehabilitation*, vol. 68 (1988), pp. 880–889.

Fast, Avital. "Low Back Pain during Pregnancy," pp. 345–351 in A. J. Cole and S. A. Herring (eds.). *Low Back Pain Handbook: A Practical Guide for the Primary Care Physician*. Hanley & Belfus, Philadelphia, 1996.

Fishman, L. M., and P. A. Zybert, "Electrophysiological Evidence of Piriformis Syndrome," *Archives of Physical Medicine and Rehabilitation*, vol. 73 (April 1992), pp. 359–364.

Forey, Peter, and Philippe Janvier. "Evolution of the Early Vertebrates," *American Scientist*, vol. 82 (1994), pp. 554–565.

Fortin, J. D., C. N. Aprill, B. Ponthieux, and J. Pier. "Sacroiliac Joint Pain Referral Maps upon Applying a New Injection/Arthrography Technique. Part II: Clinical Evaluation," *Spine*, vol. 19 (July 1994), pp. 1483–1489.

Friedlieb, O. P. "The Impact of Managed Care on the Diagnosis and Treatment of Low Back Pain: A Preliminary Report," *Journal of the American College of Medical Quality*, vol. 9, no. 1 (Spring 1994), pp. 24–29.

Giles, L. G. F. *Anatomical Basis of Low Back Pain*. Williams & Wilkins, Baltimore, 1985.

Hallin, Roger P. "Sciatic Pain and the Piriformis Muscle," *Postgraduate Medicine*, vol. 74, no. 2 (1983), pp. 69–74.

Hughes, Steven S., et al. "Extrapelvic Compression of the Sciatic Nerve," *Journal of Bone and Joint Disease*, vol. 74A, no. 10 (December 1992), pp. 1555–1558.

International Association for the Study of Pain, Subcommittee on Taxonomy, H. Merskey, chairman. "Pain Terms: A List with Definitions and Notes on Usage," pp. 249–252 in *Pain* 1979.

Jackson, C. P. "Physical Therapy for Lumbar Disc Disease," *Seminars in Spine Surgery*, vol. 1, no. 1 (1989), pp. 28–34.

Jensen, Maureen C., et al. "Magnetic Resonance Imaging of the Lumbar Spine in People without Back Pain," *New England Journal of Medicine*, vol. 331, no. 2 (July 14, 1994), pp. 69–73.

Jenkins, E. M., and D. G. Borenstein. "Exercise for the Low Back Pain Patient," *Baillieres Clinical Rheumatology*, vol. 8 (February 1994), pp. 191–197.

Keim, Hugo A., and W. H. Kirkaldy-Willis. "Low Back Pain," *Clinical Symposia* (Ciba-Geigy), vol. 32, no. 6 (1981), pp. 2–26.

Margo, K., "Diagnosis, Treatment and Prognosis in Patients with Low Back Pain," *American Family Physician*, vol. 49 (January 1994), pp. 171–179, 183–184.

Malmivaara, A., et al. "The Treatment of Acute Low Back Pain—Bed Rest, Exercises, or Ordinary Activity?" *New England Journal of Medicine*, vol. 332 (February 9, 1995), pp. 351–355.

Mixter, W. J., and J. S. Barr, "Ruptures of the Intervertebral Disc with Involvement of the Spinal Canal," *New England Journal of Medicine*, vol. 211 (1934), p. 210.

Nwuga, Vincent. *Manual Treatment of Low Back Pain*. Robert E. Krieger Publishing, Malabar, Fla., 1984.

Pace, J. B., and D. Nagle. "Piriform Syndrome," *Western Journal of Medicine*, vol. 124 (June 1976), pp. 435–439.

Parziale, J. R., T. H. Hudgins, and L. M. Fishman, "Piriformis Syndrome," *American Journal of Orthopedics*, vol. 14, (December 1996), pp. 819–823.

Porterfield, D. O., and R. J. DeRosa, *Mechanical Low Back Pain: Perspectives in Functional Anatomy*, W. B. Saunders, Philadelphia, 1991.

Saal, Joel, "Pathophysiology of Lumbar Disc Disease," unpublished paper, Daly City, Calif.

Sarno, John. *Healing Back Pain: The Mind-Body Connection*. Warner Books, New York, 1991.

Schmidt-Nielsen, Knut. *Scaling: Why Is Animal Size So Important?* Cambridge University Press, New York, 1984.

Sichlau, Michael J., James S. T. Yao, and Robert I. Vogelzang. "Transcatheter Embolectomy for the Treatment of Pelvic Congestion Syndrome," *Obstetrics and Gynecology*, vol. 83 (1994), pp. 893–896.

Stedman's Medical Dictionary, 22nd edition. Williams & Wilkins, Baltimore, 1975.

Thomas, D. C., R. W. Stones, C. M. Farquhar, and R. W. Beard, "Measurement of Pelvic Blood Flow Changes in Response to Posture in Normal Subjects and in Women with Pelvic Pain Owing to Congestion by Using a Thermal Technique," *Clinical Science,* vol. 83 (1992), pp. 55–58.

Toomey, Timothy C., Douglas Mann, Jeanne Hernandez, and Sandra Hernandez. "Psychometric Characteristics of a Brief Measure of Pain-Related Functional Impairment," *Archives of Physical Medicine and Rehabilitation,* vol. 74, (December 1993), pp. 1305–1308.

Twomey, L., and J. Taylor. "Exercise and Spinal Manipulation in the Treatment of Low Back Pain," *Spine,* vol. 20 (March 1, 1995), pp. 615–619.

Travell, Janet G., and David G. Simons. *Myofascial Pain and Dysfunction,* vols. 1 and 2. Williams & Wilkins, Baltimore, 1994.

Weinstein, J., et al. "Lumbar Disc Herniation: A Comparison of the Results of Chemonucleolysis and Open Diskectomy after Ten Years," *Journal of Bone and Joint Surgery,* vol. 68A, no. 43 (1986), pp. 43–46.

White, Augustus A. *Your Aching Back.* Simon & Schuster, New York, 1990.

White, Augustus A., and M. M. Panjabi. *Clinical Biomechanics of the Spine,* 2nd edition. Lippincott, Philadelphia, 1990.

Wiesel, S. W., et al. "Acute Low Back Pain: An Objective Analysis of Conservative Therapy," *Spine,* vol. 5 (1980), pp. 324–338.

Wiersma, C. A. G. *Invertebrate Nervous Systems: Their Significance for Mammalian Neurophysiology.* University of Chicago Press, Chicago, 1967.

Wilmore, Douglas W. "Catabolic Illness: Strategies for Enhancing Recovery," *New England Journal of Medicine,* vol. 325, no. 10 (September 5, 1991), pp. 695–702.

Index